The Handbook of Nausea and Vomiting

The Handbook of Nausea and Vomiting

General Editor:
Marvin H. Sleisenger, MD
Professor of Medicine and
Director, Cancer Research Institute
University of California, San Francisco
San Francisco, California

12 Contributors

Published in association with

Caduceus Medical Publishers

by

The Parthenon Publishing Group
New York   London

Editorial Director
John Mesevage

Managing Editor
Stu Chapman

Associate Editor
Andrea Lazarus

Assistant Editor
Beth Beyer

Indexer
Margaret Jarpey

Design Director
Michael McClain

Production Director
Laura Carlson

Publishers
Paul Henrici
Glenn Moser

Printed in the United States of America

Published in association with
Caduceus Medical Publishers, Inc.
One Fenwood Drive
Pawling, NY 12564, USA,

by

The Parthenon Publishing Group
One Blue Hill Plaza
Pearl River, NY 10965, USA
and
30 Blades Court, London, England

ISBN   1-85070-528-3

Contributors

Robert W. Baloh, MD
Professor
Department of Neurology and
Division of Head and Neck Surgery
  (Otolaryngology)
UCLA School of Medicine
Los Angeles, California

Burton S. Epstein, MD
Seymour Alpert Professor
Department of Anesthesia
George Washington University
Washington, DC

Paul J. Hesketh, MD
Associate Professor of Medicine
Boston University School of Medicine
Boston, Massachusetts

Susan Kim, PharmD
Poison Information Specialist
San Francisco Bay Area
  Regional Poison Control Center
San Francisco General Hospital
Associate Clinical Professor of Pharmacy
University of California, San Francisco
San Francisco, California

Tekoa King, CNM, MPH
Assistant Professor
Department of Obstetrics, Gynecology,
  and Reproductive Sciences
University of California, San Francisco
San Francisco, California

Kenneth L. Koch, MD
Professor of Medicine
Gastroenterology Division
University Hospital,
The Pennsylvania State University
Hershey, Pennsylvania

Alan D. Miller, PhD
Associate Professor
Laboratory of Neurophysiology
The Rockefeller University
New York, New York

Gary R. Morrow, PhD
Director, Behavioral Medicine Unit
University of Rochester Cancer Center
Associate Professor of Oncology in Psychiatry
University of Rochester School of Medicine
  and Dentistry
Rochester, New York

Kent R. Olson, MD
Medical Director
San Francisco Bay Area
  Regional Poison Control Center
San Francisco General Hospital
Associate Clinical Professor of Medicine
University of California, San Francisco
San Francisco, California

Julian T. Parer, MD, PhD
Professor
Department of Obstetrics, Gynecology,
  and Reproductive Sciences
University of California, San Francisco
San Francisco, California

Sidney F. Phillips, MD
Professor of Medicine
Gastroenterology Research Unit
Mayo Clinic and Medical School
Rochester, Minnesota

T. J. Priestman, MD
Consultant Clinical Oncologist
The Royal Hospital
Wolverhampton
United Kingdom

Preface

The purpose of this book is to help clinicians better understand the relationship of nausea and vomiting to various clinical diseases and disorders and to treat these symptoms more effectively. As a handbook, it is a practical, easy-to-use reference to current medical opinion, providing guidelines to improve clinical decision making.

Each of the twelve editors has extensively studied nausea and vomiting within a special field and has published widely in the peer-reviewed medical literature. Their expertise, based on the thousands of patients they have studied in diverse clinical settings, gives the book a tremendous breadth of clinical relevance. Despite the diversity of their clinical experience and the specialized focus of their studies, their observations and analyses often are interrelated. I am impressed by this observation, which emphasizes that nausea and vomiting are best understood from a perspective shared by all of these investigators.

The mechanisms underlying nausea and vomiting have long been poorly understood. Only recently have studies adequately addressed misconceptions that prevented more effective management. One of the misconceptions concerns the existence of a "vomiting center," a discrete anatomical entity that controls the emetic response. The current view is that a vomiting center—at least as a definable anatomic entity—has not been found. Throughout the book, however, reference is made to the vomiting center, a term that is used advisedly and from a pharmacologic rather than an anatomic point of view.

Although investigators have not precisely located a vomiting center, a great deal more is now known about the neural pathways involved in nausea and vomiting. These pathways appear to be active in a variety of settings—postoperative recovery, cancer chemotherapy and irradiation, obstetrics, and treatment of gastrointestinal disorders. The contributors' perspectives in each of these and other areas make clear the multifactorial nature of nausea and vomiting, particularly some of the nuances of brain-gut interaction.

Regardless of the circumstances, similar mechanisms often underlie the emetic response.

I find this multifactorial etiology exciting because of its potential implications for tailoring therapy for specific patients. In few areas is this more apparent than in cancer chemotherapy and in postoperative management, where awareness of the role of serotonin receptors has dramatically revised strategies to prevent emesis. A broad choice of therapies, utilizing combinations of antiemetic agents, is now available and offers hope to patients whose clinical course would be more complicated because of nausea and vomiting.

Despite the progress toward more effective treatment, many patients remain refractory to antiemetic medications. In some cases—such as the anticipatory nausea and vomiting associated with chemotherapy—we are reminded how much we need to learn before these symptoms can be controlled or even significantly reduced.

By chronicling the progress we have made in preventing nausea and vomiting and promoting a better understanding of these symptoms, perhaps *The Handbook of Nausea and Vomiting* will serve a twofold purpose: helping readers confront and manage a problem common to every clinical practice, and encouraging more ambitious research to improve the quality of patient care.

Marvin H. Sleisenger, MD
Editor
Professor of Medicine and
Director, Cancer Research Institute
University of California, San Francisco
San Francisco, California

Table of Contents

CHAPTER 10   143

Nausea or Vomiting Associated with Poisoning or Drug Overdose

Susan Kim and Kent R. Olson

Index   163

Neuroanatomy and Physiology

Alan D. Miller, PhD

The essential neuronal circuitry for producing vomiting, apart from sensory inputs and motor outputs, is located within the medulla of the brain stem.[1] The concept of a "vomiting center" originated with early experiments in animal models in the 1940s. This center was envisioned to be an anatomically distinct area in the brain stem that received input from all emetic sensory sources and initiated the emetic response through its connections to various effector motor nuclei. Despite numerous references to the vomiting center in the literature and the widely held perception that it has been identified, the existence of such an anatomically well-localized structure remains controversial. Convincing evidence is still lacking, and pinpointing the vomiting center remains an elusive goal of neurophysiologic research.

In addition to the brain stem, other regions of the brain can be involved in initiation of vomiting under certain circumstances, such as in psychogenic vomiting. Electrical stimulation of certain rostral brain regions can lead to vomiting,[2,3] undoubtedly via excitation of medullary structures.

Our understanding of the neuroanatomy and physiology underlying nausea and vomiting has improved in the last ten years. We have a better understanding of the kinds of sensory input received, the neurotransmitter receptor subtypes involved, and the neuronal pathways utilized to transmit output. For example, the role of the abdominal visceral nerves, particularly the vagus and splanchnic nerves, has been clarified. **(See Chapters 5 and 9.)**

The Area Postrema as a Chemoreceptor Trigger Zone for Vomiting

The concept of the area postrema as a central chemoreceptor trigger zone for vomiting was developed approximately 40 years ago.[4,5] The area postrema is thought to be the major central detector of circulating toxins. Located on the floor of the caudal end of the fourth ventricle, it lies outside the conventional blood-brain barrier (Fig 1).[4,5] Apart from its role in emesis,

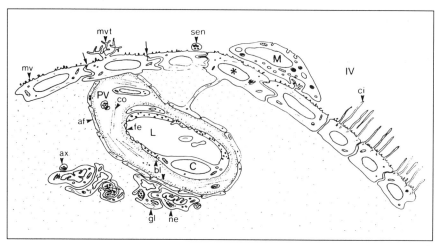

Fig 1. Cytologic features of the area postrema (AP). The ependymal cells overlying the nucleus have variable numbers of microvilli (mv), and one bears a microvillous tuft (mvt). Arrows indicate the apical borders between these cells, where specialized intercellular junctions are found. A supraependymal neuronal (axonal) element (sen) is illustrated next to a supraependymal macrophage (M). Adjacent ventricular ependymal cells are ciliated (ci), unlike those of the AP itself. One of the AP ependymal cells (*) has a basal cytoplasmic extension that forms, with other such cellular profiles (af), a partial ensheathment of a perivascular space (PV) around a capillary (C); L indicates its lumen. Within the space are found collagen bundles (co), fibroblasts, other cytoplasmic elements (axonal varicosities), and internal and external basal laminae (bl). A pericyte can be seen between the internal basal lamina and the endothelium of the capillary. The endothelial cell is fenestrated (fe). A few glial cells (gl) and neuronal somata (ne) are illustrated, as well as axonal varicosities (ax). Intravascular space is also shown (IV). (From Leslie RA. Comparative aspects of the area postrema: fine-structural considerations help to determine its function. *Cell Molec Neurobiol.* 1986;6:95–120.)

the area postrema has also been implicated in such functions as conditioned taste aversion, control of food intake, fluid homeostasis, and cardiovascular control.[4,5] The area postrema is an important site for sensory input. Its presumed role in the pathophysiology of nausea and vomiting is based to a large extent on evidence demonstrating that lesions of the area postrema prevent vomiting induced by many emetic drugs.[4] In addition, electrophysiology studies have shown that neurons in the area postrema are excited by local application of a number of emetic substances.[6]

Ablation of the area postrema may not prevent vomiting in certain situations. Substances that persist in inducing vomiting despite lesions in the area postrema include naloxone[7] and the serotonin-3 receptor agonist phenylbiguanide (PBG).[8] In addition, area postrema lesions do not prevent vomiting induced by electrical stimulation of abdominal vagal afferents[8] or, despite earlier reports, by motion.[4] It is still uncertain whether the area postrema, as opposed to other nearby sensory pathways, plays a significant role in radiation-induced vomiting.[4]

As reviewed by Leslie,[5] the major inputs to the area postrema arise from the trigeminal (V), glossopharyngeal (IX), and vagus (X) cranial nerves, dorsomedial and paraventricular hypothalamic subnuclei, the nucleus of the solitary tract, and the pontine lateral parabrachial nucleus. Widespread efferent projections from the area postrema have been described in the lateral parabrachial nucleus, dorsal portion of solitary nucleus, dorsal motor vagal nucleus, nucleus ambiguous, ventrolateral medullary catecholaminergic A1 cell group, mesencephalic nucleus of the trigeminal nerve, dorsal spinal trigeminal nucleus, paratrigeminal nucleus, and region of the cerebellar vermis.[5] Thus, the area postrema does not serve simply as a relay to a still elusive vomiting center; it seems situated to play a more complex role in emesis and perhaps other autonomic functions.

The Search for the Vomiting Center

The Original Model

Borison and Wang[9,10] developed the concept of a vomiting center in the dorsolateral reticular formation on the basis of studies of cats and dogs showing that vomiting can be produced by electrically stimulating a region of the brain stem of unanesthetized, decerebrate cats and that large lesions in this region interfered with a dog's response to emetic agents. Subsequent research refined earlier concepts, elucidated other mechanisms involved in the emetic response, and proposed new models.

In 1983, for example, we attempted to repeat the electrical stimulation studies from which the concept of a vomiting center was derived, hoping to identify a more localized region where vomiting could be evoked.[11] We were unable to elicit readily reproducible vomiting.[11] We argued that if a well-localized vomiting center existed in this region of the brain stem, its activation by electrical stimulation should produce vomiting reliably.

Electrical stimulation and lesions of the brain stem affect not only cell bodies but also axons of passage. This probably explains the results of earlier research, which may have affected vagal sensory afferents, area postrema efferents, and/or premotor outputs. Electrical stimulation of the abdominal vagus nerve, for example, can reproducibly evoke vomiting at short latencies.[12] Vomiting can also be elicited by stimulation along the vagal sensory input pathway within the brain stem.[13]

The Botzinger Complex

A recent investigation sought to clarify the location of the "pattern generator for the emetic act" by studying retching and vomiting in decerebrate, paralyzed dogs.[13] Large lesions in the lateral portion of the brain stem at the level of the retrofacial nucleus abolished vomiting, which is consistent with our findings in cats. These investigators concluded that the region of the Botzinger complex near the retrofacial nucleus contains the central pattern generator for vomiting.[13] Although intriguing, the results do not justify this conclusion. As discussed by Miller,[1] demonstration of the existence of a pattern generator akin to a vomiting center requires more compelling data. Investigators would need to:

(1) determine that the effects of lesion and stimulation were due to effects on neuronal cell bodies rather than on axons passing through the region.

(2) better localize the effective site within the confines of the lesioned area.

(3) ensure that the results were not due to perturbation of premotor and motor-output circuitry.

(4) identify neurons in this region that display the appropriate discharge and that connect to function in a way compatible with a vomiting center.

Premotor neurons in this region are involved in generating the pattern of respiratory muscle discharge during vomiting.[1] However, this premotor circuitry is unlikely to function as a vomiting center because it probably does not project to all the necessary effector nuclei that require activation to produce vomiting-related phenomena. In this context, it is important to note that instead of monitoring the entire act of vomiting, Fukuda and Koga[13] used a characteristic pattern of respiratory muscle nerve discharge. Thus, it is unknown whether lesions in the Botzinger region also abolish other components (e.g., gastrointestinal).

Even though no study has met the four above criteria, the region around the retrofacial nucleus may be a promising site for further investigation into the neuronal mechanisms that coordinate vomiting.

Other Models

Another line of research seems to be moving further away from the concept of a vomiting center where control arises from a central "black box." It may be time to more seriously consider other models that could serve as the basis for experimental work. Two new models have been proposed as alternatives to the traditional concept of a vomiting center. The first suggests that vomiting may be produced by the sequential activation of a series of effector nuclei, rather than by the coordination of these motor nuclei in parallel by a vomiting center.[14] This model suggests that the vomiting center is difficult to locate because it is not a discrete entity but rather the higher function of an ensemble of separate effector nuclei.[14]

The other new model concerns a paraventricular system of nuclei, defined by their connections with the area postrema and with each other.[15] Lawes proposed that these nuclei may account for most of the phenomena associated with nausea and vomiting and thus may more closely approximate the vomiting center that has eluded the grasp of investigators.[15]

Therapeutic Implications

It remains to be seen whether these models more accurately reflect the mechanisms involved in nausea and vomiting or whether they, too, could succumb to new theories that may more accurately describe the pathophysiology. Whatever the differences in these models, the ultimate test of their worth is whether they will contribute toward the development of therapy that can more effectively control nausea and vomiting. Approaching this problem from different avenues, investigators have sought to more precisely characterize the cells involved in the emetic response, identify transmitters within that complex, and develop antagonists to certain subtypes of transmitter receptors.

A prime example of this line of research is studies assessing the role of serotonin-3 (5-HT$_3$) receptors in producing vomiting. Antagonists to 5-HT$_3$ receptors are showing promise in combating vomiting induced by cancer chemotherapy **(see Chapter 9)**. This drug class also appears to be effective in preventing or reducing radiation-induced vomiting.

Recent studies have sought to identify the locations of 5-HT$_3$ receptors involved in initiating vomiting by cutting visceral afferents or by creating lesions in the area postrema. The threshold of vomiting induced by the 5-HT$_3$ receptor agonist PBG was greatly increased by section of the vagus and splanchnic nerves in cats.[8] Lesions of the area postrema abolished vomiting in response to cisplatin but had no apparent effect on vomiting induced by PBG or by electrical stimulation of abdominal vagal afferents.[8] These findings are consistent with another recent study indicating that cisplatin acts via multiple mechanisms involving both activation of the nucleus of the solitary tract via visceral afferents and independent activation of the area postrema.[16]

These results support the idea that a given stimulus may produce vomiting by parallel mechanisms; however, one pathway may be predominant for a specific stimulus or species.[17] In contrast, earlier models of emesis were relatively simplistic, postulating that nausea and vomiting were triggered as input to a well-localized coordinating center. We may need to consider multiple pathways as part of a more complex pathophysiology than earlier research suggested.

The Physiology of Vomiting

Nausea and vomiting are components of the body's defense system to protect against the accidental ingestion of toxins. These events are also responses to additional stimuli, including psychogenic stimuli, those affecting the vestibular system (as in the case of motion sickness), and those that cause sickness in pregnancy.

The oral expulsion of upper gut contents is produced by the coordinated action of the respiratory muscles and gastrointestinal tract. Prodromal changes, such as licking, salivation, pallor, and changes in heart rate, may also occur.[18]

Gastrointestinal components. Prior to vomiting, toxins are confined to the stomach by relaxation of the proximal stomach and by a major contraction moving retrograde from the small intestine to the stomach.[19] Lang and Sarna[19] suggested that an important function of the retrograde giant contraction may be to buffer and dilute the acidic stomach contents with intestinal or pancreaticobiliary secretions. Vomiting is also accompanied by relaxation of the lower esophageal sphincter and longitudinal shortening of the esophagus.[19] **(See Chapter 6.)**

Respiratory muscle components. During the retching phase, successive waves of abdominal and diaphragmatic co-contractions cause large pressure swings in the thorax and abdomen.[20] The retching phase is followed by an expulsive phase, in which the high positive pressure in both the thorax and abdomen is accompanied by relaxation of the inner hiatal part of the diaphragm.[21,22] Abdominal muscle activity is prolonged during expulsion, with respect to both diaphragmatic activity and abdominal discharge during the retching phase.[23] The external intercostal (inspiratory) muscles also co-contract with the diaphragm and abdominal muscles during vomiting. In contrast, the internal intercostal (expiratory) muscles contract out of phase with these other muscles and generate little or no positive thoracic pressure (Fig 2).[20]

The relaxation of the periesophageal portion of the diaphragm presumably facilitates rostral movement of gastric contents. This relaxation is greatest during expulsion; however, some reduction in activity also occurs during retching. Periesophageal relaxation during vomiting does not depend on a reflex arising from movement of vomitus within the esophagus and is part of the central motor program for vomiting.[21]

Muscles of the upper airway protect the nasopharynx and trachea by raising the soft palate and closing the glottis. Closure muscles of the glottis discharge in phase with bursts of diaphragmatic and abdominal nerve discharge during vomiting, while the glottis opener remains silent.[24,25] Also active dur-

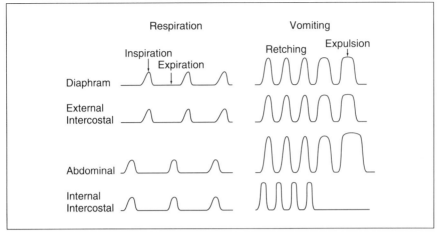

Fig 2. Activity of the major respiratory muscles during respiration and vomiting. Diaphragm and abdominal muscle data are from numerous laboratories. Intercostal muscle data during vomiting are according to McCarthy and Borison (1974). (From Miller AD. Respiratory muscle control during vomiting. *Can J Physio Pharmaco.* 1990;68:237–241. Modified from Miller and Tan [1987], with permission.)

ing these bursts are the genioglossus, which causes protrusion of the tongue, and stylopharyngeus, which dilates and elevates the pharynx. The digastricus, which depresses the lower jaw, is active throughout the retching and expulsion phases.[24] Following expulsion, bursts of oropharyngeal nerve discharge correspond to the buccopharyngeal stage of swallowing.[24]

To what extent are the brain stem neurons that are involved in respiration also involved in vomiting? Respiratory muscles are controlled in part during vomiting by some of the same propriobulbar and bulbospinal respiratory neurons involved in control during breathing. In addition to excitatory inputs, neuroinhibition is also important in shaping the discharge of premotor and motor outputs during vomiting. However, it is uncertain which neurons are responsible for activating phrenic and external intercostal motoneurons during vomiting.[1,23] An improved understanding of the brain stem circuitry responsible for respiratory muscle control during vomiting is important to delineate the pathways and transmitters involved.

Conclusion

A vomiting center within the medulla of the brain stem has long been thought to be an essential element in the neuroanatomy and physiology of nausea and vomiting. Since the 1940s, investigators have believed that such a center is responsible for coordinating emetogenic sensory input and projecting it to motor output nuclei, thereby triggering emesis. This concept, however, is evolving, as new studies are questioning whether such a well-localized area exists.

The area postrema, often referred to as a "chemoreceptor trigger zone," is an important site for sensory input and can play a key role in evoking nausea and vomiting, but its ablation may not prevent vomiting in certain situations. The abdominal vagus nerve, vestibular apparatus, and rostral brain regions can also be important for inducing vomiting under certain conditions. Recent research has proposed new models of the emetic response, which rely less on the concept of a vomiting center per se and suggest that multiple pathways may be involved in the pathophysiology. The effectiveness of newly developed antagonists to serotonin-3 receptors supports the concept that certain subtypes of neurotransmitter receptors play a role in initiating vomiting.

Physiologically, vomiting is a motor act, resulting primarily from the coordinated action of the respiratory muscles and gastrointestinal tract. Some of the brain stem neurons involved in respiratory muscle control during breathing are also active during vomiting. Further study of the brain stem circuitry is needed to determine how various pathways and neurotransmitters produce vomiting.

References

1. Miller AD. Physiology of brain stem emetic circuitry. In: Bianchi AL, Grelot L, Miller AD, King GL, eds. *Colloque INSERM*. Montrouge, France: John Libbey Eurotext Ltd.; 1992;223:41–50.

2. Hess WR. The functional organization of the diencephalon. In: Hughes JR, ed. *Mechanisms and Control of Emesis*. New York: Grune and Stratton; 1957.

3. Robinson BW, Mishkin M. Alimentary responses to forebrain stimulation in monkeys. *Exp Brain Res*. 1968;4:330–366.

4. Borison HL. Area postrema: chemoreceptor circumventricular organ of the medulla oblongata. *Prog Neurobiol*. 1989;32:351–390.

5. Leslie RA. Comparative aspects of the area postrema: fine-structural considerations help to determine its function. *Cell Molec Neurobiol*. 1986;6:95–120.

6. Carpenter DO, Briggs DB, Knox AP. Excitation of area postrema neurons by transmitters, peptides, and cyclic nucleotides. *J Neurophysiol*. 1988;59:358–369.

7. Costello DJ, Borison HL. Naloxone antagonizes narcotic self-blockade of emesis in the cat. *J Pharmacol Exper Ther*. 1977;203:222–230.

8. Miller AD, Nonaka S. Mechanisms of vomiting induced by serotonin-3 receptor agonists in the cat: effect of vagotomy, splanchnicectomy or area postrema lesion. *J Pharmacol Exper Ther*. 1992;260:509–517.

9. Borison HL, Wang SC. Functional localization of central coordinating mechanism for emesis in cat. *J Neurophysiol*. 1949;12:305–313.

10. Wang SC, Borison HL. The vomiting center: its destruction by radon implantation in dog medulla oblongata. *Am J Physiol.* 1951;166:712–717.

11. Miller AD, Wilson VJ. "Vomiting center" reanalyzed: an electrical stimulation study. *Brain Res.* 1983;270:154–158.

12. Miller AD, Tan LK, Suzuki I. Control of abdominal and expiratory intercostal muscle activity during vomiting: role of ventral respiratory group expiratory neurons. *J Neurophysiol.* 1987;57:1854–1866.

13. Fukuda H, Koga T. The Botzinger complex as the pattern generator for retching and vomiting in the dog. *Neurosci Res.* 1991;12:471–485.

14. Davis CJ, Harding RK, Leslie RA, Andrews PLR. The organisation of vomiting as a protective reflex. In: Davis CJ, Lake-Bakaar GV, Grahame-Smith DG, eds. *Nausea and Vomiting: Mechanisms and Treatment.* Berlin, Germany: Springer-Verlag; 1986:65–75.

15. Lawes INC. The central connections of the area postrema define the paraventricular system involved in antinoxious behaviors. In: Kucharczyk J, Stewart DJ, Miller AD, eds. *Nausea and Vomiting: Recent Research and Clinical Advances.* Boca Raton, Fla: CRC Press; 1991:77–101.

16. Reynolds DJM, Barber NA, Grahame-Smith DG, Leslie RA. Cisplatin-evoked induction of c-fos protein in the brainstem of the ferret: the effect of cervical vagotomy and the antiemetic 5-HT$_3$ receptor antagonist granisetron (BRL 43694). *Brain Res.* 1991;565:231–236.

17. Harding RK. Concepts and conflicts in the mechanism of emesis. *Can J Physiol Pharmacol.* 1990;68:218–220.

18. Andrews PLR, Hawthorn J. The neurophysiology of vomiting. *Bailliere's Clin Gastroenterol.* 1988;2:141–168.

19. Lang IM, Sarna SK. Motor and myoelectric activity associated with vomiting, regurgitation, and nausea. In: Wood JD, ed. *Handbook of Physiology: The Gastrointestinal System I, Motility and Circulation.* Bethesda, Md: Bethesda, Md, Physiological Society; 1989:1179–1198.

20. McCarthy LE, Borison HL. Respiratory mechanics of vomiting in decerebrate cats. *Am J Physiol.* 1974;226:738–743.

21. Miller AD, Lakos SF, Tan LK. Central motor program for relaxation of periesophageal diaphragm during the expulsive phase of vomiting. *Brain Res.* 1988;456:367–370.

22. Monges H, Salducci J, Naudy B. Dissociation between the electrical activity of the diaphragmatic dome and crura muscular fibers during esophageal distention, vomiting and eructation: an electromyographic study in the dog. *J Physiol.* (Paris) 1978;74:541–554.

23. Miller AD. Vomiting: its respiratory components. In: Speck DF, Dekin MS, Revelette WR, Frazier DT, eds. *Respiratory Control: Central and Peripheral Mechanisms.* Lexington, Ky: University Press; 1992:207–210.

24. Grelot L, Barillot JC, Bianchi AL. Activity of respiratory-related oropharyngeal and laryngeal motoneurons during fictive vomiting in the decerebrate cat. *Brain Res.* 1990;513:101–105.

25. Hukuhara T, Okada H, Yamagami M. On the behavior of the respiratory muscles during vomiting. *Acta Med Okayama.* 1957;11:117–125.

9

CHAPTER 2

Psychological Aspects of Nausea and Vomiting: Anticipation of Chemotherapy

Gary R. Morrow, PhD

Nausea and vomiting in anticipation of chemotherapy remains one of the most persistent and troublesome complications limiting efforts to control or cure cancer. Anticipatory nausea and vomiting (ANV) is highly prevalent and refractory to antiemetic therapy. Although estimates vary widely, ranging from 18% to 63%, a meta-analysis of 29 studies with 2,452 patients suggests that the overall prevalence of ANV is about 25%, approximately one third as prevalent as posttreatment nausea and vomiting.[1]

Despite the scope of the problem and the need to predict which patients are at risk, the etiology of ANV is not clearly understood. The poor characterization of its causes is partly due to the widely held perception that patients who develop this complication are psychologically disturbed. Only recently have studies begun to pinpoint characteristics associated with occurrence of anticipatory side effects and to develop models that delineate the etiology (Fig 1).[2] These models could improve our understanding of mechanisms involved in ANV and enable us to predict with some accuracy which patients will develop such complications. The improved understanding also could lead to more efficient allocation of clinical resources and more effective preventive interventions in high-risk subsets of patients.

Extensions from theory and animal research into the applied clinical arena are often inexact, but it appears that anticipatory nausea is a learned response.[3] Learning theory is one of three major areas of research in determining how various factors contribute to the development of anticipatory side effects. The other research areas are measurements of individual differences, and clinical observations.

No study has ever reported ANV without previous posttreatment nausea and vomiting. As a corollary, the severity of posttreatment symptoms is likely to be related to the severity of ANV. Delayed nausea and vomiting, a phenomenon that is not clearly understood, may also be

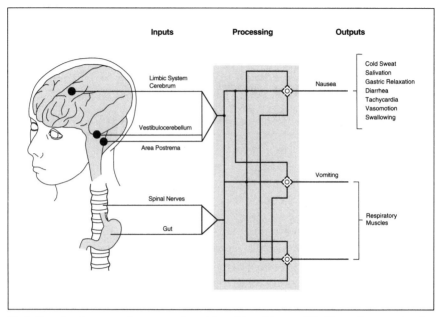

| Inputs | Processing | Outputs |

Fig 1. Functional aspects of nausea and vomiting. (From Morrow GR. Chemotherapy-related nausea and vomiting: etiology and management. *Cancer.* **1989;39:89–104.)**

related to ANV. For example, patients undergoing chemotherapy treatment may experience emesis after a 24-hour symptom-free period following chemotherapy treatment.

Models of Etiology

The most promising theory of how AN develops closely follows the principles of learning.[4] There are basically two models of learning: *operant* and *classical.*

The operant model suggests that behavior develops and continues because it is reinforced. This model may be appropriate in many settings, but it is suspect when applied to ANV. The extension of the operant model further suggests that the patient receives some reward for nausea and vomiting behavior. Although nausea and vomiting are attended to by those responsible for treatment, it stretches credibility that someone would continue such behavior for the meager reinforcement provided.[4] The high prevalence of ANV casts further doubt on the validity of this model.

The classical learning model is a more reasonable explanation of the sequence of events in ANV. In this model, a previously neutral stimulus (or

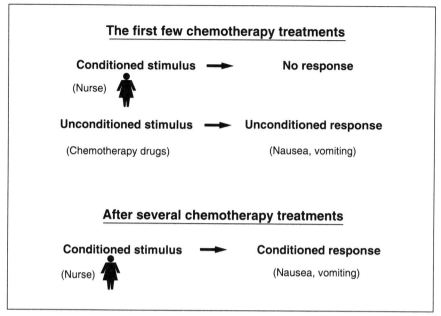

Fig 2. Conditioning model of how anticipatory side effects develop. (From Morrow GR, Dobkin PL. Anticipatory nausea and vomiting in cancer patients undergoing chemotherapy treatment: prevalence, etiology, and behaviorial interventions. *Clin Psych Rev.* 1988;8:517–556.)

"conditioned stimulus") that is part of treatment (such as the nurse or clinic environment) is associated with the administration of chemotherapy that causes posttreatment nausea and vomiting ("unconditioned response").[3] During repeated treatments ("conditioning trials"), the conditioned stimulus begins to elicit ANV as a conditioned response (Fig 2).[4]

Data tend to support the classical learning model, and no data have contradicted it.[5] The learning principles governing the development of ANV are more specifically characterized this way:

• **Course of development.** Classically conditioned responses develop only after one or more pairings of the conditioned stimulus with the unconditioned response.[1] The greater the number of pairings, the greater the likelihood that the conditioned response will develop. This view is supported by clinical observations that ANV is virtually never seen before patients have undergone a number of chemotherapy treatments ("conditioning trials") and have experienced posttreatment nausea and vomiting. Evidence also suggests that as the number of chemotherapy courses increases, so does the percentage of patients who develop ANV (Fig 3).[4] These findings are consistent with the theory that a response grows stronger with the number of conditioning trials.[4]

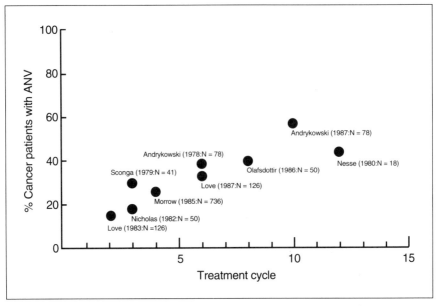

Fig 3. Prevalence of anticipatory nausea and vomiting (ANV) versus number of chemotherapy treatments. (From Morrow GR, Dobkin PL. Anticipatory nausea and vomiting in cancer patients undergoing chemotherapy treatment: prevalence, etiology, and behavioral interventions. *Clin Psych Rev.* 1988;8:517–556.)

- **Stimulus generalization.** As treatment continues, another principle of learning theory, concerned with generalizing a stimulus, becomes relevant. In this case, a response may be elicited by a stimulus similar to the original conditioned stimulus.[4] In a clinical setting, it is not uncommon for patients to report nausea when they see the clinic nurse who administers their drugs; later, after a few more chemotherapy treatments, the sight of any clinic nurse elicits nausea.[6]

- **Intensity of unconditioned response.** Classical conditioning theory also states that the intensity of an unconditioned response affects the development of a conditioned response. When applied to ANV, this means that the severity of posttreatment nausea and vomiting after the first course of treatment (unconditioned response) would be related to the development of ANV (conditioned response). Eight studies confirm that the severity of posttreatment nausea and vomiting is significantly associated with the development of ANV, and increased severity of the initial response correlates with a higher incidence of ANV.[4]

- **Higher-order conditioning.** In addition to these relationships, ANV may be triggered by other stimuli as a result of higher-order conditioning. Through higher-order conditioning, neutral stimuli can elicit a conditioned response if paired with a conditioned stimulus. Although a higher-order conditioned stimulus does not typically elicit a conditioned response as intensely or as frequently as does the conditioned stimulus, it is a potent factor. In support of this view is the observation that as a patient approaches the treatment center, the intensity of ANV tends to increase.[8] Stimuli, such as the hospital parking lot, which are associated with the patient's arrival and imminent treatment session are paired with conditioned stimuli such as the oncology nurse or clinic odors in higher-order conditioning.[4] Over time, an association among these stimuli is formed, and ANV becomes the overt behavioral manifestation.

The interplay of these factors in provoking ANV is evident in a study by Dobkin et al[8] in which patients were asked where they were when their anticipatory symptoms began. Sixteen patients indicated their home, three reported becoming ill while traveling to the clinic, five identified the clinic, and three reported other locations. Patients disclosed that visualizing needle insertions, and olfactory cues, including the smell of the clinic, preceded development of anticipatory complications, thereby lending circumstantial support to the theory that ANV is based on a learned response. Although no carefully controlled studies conclusively demonstrate that ANV associated with chemotherapy is unequivocally a result of learning, converging lines of indirect evidence strongly support such a view.[4]

At least two characteristics of ANV, however, are not entirely consistent with the classical conditioning model: the relatively long interval between the unconditioned stimulus (initial administration of chemotherapy drugs) and the unconditioned response (posttreatment nausea and vomiting), and the intermittent nature of the conditioned response. In classical conditioning, the interval between the unconditioned stimulus and the unconditioned response is typically seconds, or possibly minutes; in the chemotherapy setting, the interval is generally hours. This has led to speculation that ANV may be as consistent with a learned taste-aversion model as with the cognitive model of classical conditioning.[9] The intermittent nature of ANV in some patients is also somewhat at variance with a classical conditioning model.[4] Anecdotal evidence suggests that patients do not invariably develop ANV, possibly because the conditioned stimulus is not present prior to each chemotherapy treatment. For example, a nurse who is part of the conditioned stimulus may not be present at each treatment session. Because ANV does not conform precisely with classical conditioning theory, future studies are needed to determine how it can be best explained by various learning models.

Anxiety Model

Among other viewpoints proposed to explain how psychological processes may cause anticipatory side effects, the anxiety model has attracted the most interest. Anxiety potentially could be related to anticipatory side effects in four ways: (1) anticipatory nausea causes pretreatment anxiety; (2) pretreatment anxiety causes anticipatory nausea; (3) anticipatory nausea and pretreatment anxiety are both caused by posttreatment nausea; and (4) pretreatment anxiety facilitates the conditioning process of anticipatory side effects.[4] Although some data support each of these potential explanations, scientific evaluation in a clinical setting is impossible. Evidence suggests that increased anxiety may precede the initial ANV symptoms, but one cannot assume that anxiety causes anticipatory symptoms.[10] The role of anxiety may be more convoluted. Anxiety may be heightened following a particular chemotherapy treatment and, in turn, the increased anxiety may increase posttreatment nausea and vomiting. Similarly, the increased posttreatment nausea and vomiting may heighten susceptibility to conditioning on the next chemotherapy cycle as part of a circular process.[4] Some degree of anxiety probably facilitates conditioning by alerting or sensitizing the patient, as does anxiety associated with cardiac arrhythmias.

Our study involving 299 patients measured anxiety at each chemotherapy cycle as a constellation of symptoms (alteration in appetite, sweating, etc) and as psychological mood.[11] Both types of assessment were used because several symptoms commonly reported for anxiety may also be side effects of chemotherapy, irrespective of anxiety. A significant association was found between anxiety based on patient symptoms and subsequent development of ANV. When anxiety was assessed as a mood, it was not found to be related to subsequent development of anticipatory side effects during the first five chemotherapy cycles. Furthermore, symptom-based measures of anxiety were correlated with development of anticipatory side effects not only at baseline but also during treatment.

Increased anxiety may play a pivotal role in raising the probability of anticipatory effects with subsequent treatment. Heightened anxiety following the second chemotherapy treatment compared with the first session would potentiate the development of ANV on the third treatment. This was true to a certain extent in our study. Patients with the greatest increase in anxiety for their second chemotherapy treatment as compared with their initial treatment had a higher incidence of ANV prior to their third therapy session than had patients with a lesser increase in anxiety. But this trend did not persist for the fourth or fifth treatment.[1]

An intriguing question addressed by other studies is the point during a course of chemotherapy when anxiety becomes a potent factor. How many treatment sessions are required before anxiety levels cross an apparent threshold and begin to influence ANV? In prospective study of 126 patients undergoing chemotherapy (94 for breast cancer and 32 for malignant lymphoma), 38% developed ANV. Patients who experienced anxiety during injections were significantly more likely to develop ANV than nonanxious patients.[12] The association between anxiety and anticipatory nausea was not statistically significant during the first two chemotherapy cycles, but it became significant by the sixth cycle. Time frame was also relevant in another study[13] that investigated different patterns of infusion-related anxiety and posttreatment nausea prior to the onset of anticipatory side effects. Patients were divided into two groups: early onset (ANV prior to chemotherapy cycle 7), and late onset (ANV followed chemotherapy cycle 7). Anxiety appeared to contribute to the development of ANV only in the late-onset group.

Clinical Characteristics and Susceptibility to ANV

Two major conclusions have emerged from studies examining anticipatory side effects: (1) the response is most probably classically conditioned in some way; and (2) susceptibility is determined by more than one variable.[5] We examined the ability of eight clinical characteristics (Table 1) to predict anticipatory side effects[5] and found that significantly more patients with four or more of these characteristics had developed ANV by the fourth chemotherapy treatment. The eight features were:

(1) Nausea and/or vomiting after the *last* chemotherapy session.
(2) Nausea after the first chemotherapy treatment described as "moderate," "severe," or "intolerable."
(3) Vomiting after first chemotherapy treatment described as "moderate," "severe," or "intolerable."
(4) Age less than 50 years.
(5) Susceptibility to motion sickness.
(6) Generalized weakness following treatment.
(7) Sweating following treatment.
(8) Feeling warm or hot after treatment.

The significant roles played by age and susceptibility to motion sickness support the view that the etiology of anticipatory side effects may not be based solely on learning. Susceptibility to motion sickness suggests that the vestibular apparatus may be independently involved in the development of ANV. A common model for motion sickness is the mismatch in sensory cues **(see Chapter 4)**. Chemotherapy probably alters the patient's perception and integration of sensory experience. Some chemotherapeutic

Table 1. Patient Characteristics Associated With the Development of Anticipatory Nausea and Vomiting

Age less than 50

Nausea/vomiting after last chemotherapy session

Posttreatment nausea described as "moderate", "severe", or "intolerable"

Posttreatment vomiting described as "moderate", "severe", or "intolerable"

Feeling warm or hot all over after last chemotherapy session

Susceptibility to motion sickness

Sweating after last chemotherapy session

Generalized weakness after last chemotherapy session

From Morrow GR. Chemotherapy-related nausea and vomiting: etiology and management. *Cancer.* 1989;39:89–104.

drugs influence the expression of fine motor coordination, which in turn could influence eye movement and the ability to track objects smoothly. The discrepancy between what a person expects to see and what is actually seen might create the type of mismatch that provokes motion-induced symptoms like nausea.[5] Although this theory is tantalizing, little evidence suggests that susceptibility to motion sickness influences ANV by heightening the unconditioned response of posttreatment nausea. Further studies are needed to elucidate how susceptibility to motion sickness relates to various learning models.

Additional study is also needed to explore the influence of age and its possible indirect effect on learning. Perhaps because younger cancer patients have less experience with medical treatment and sensations, sights, and experiences than do older patients, their lack of familiarity may strengthen the unconditioned response. Younger patients may perceive the unconditioned response of postchemotherapy nausea more keenly than older patients and may become more cognitively aware of various stimuli and responses. Such heightened awareness may promote the conditioning process.

While the contribution of age and susceptibility to motion sickness require additional analysis to determine their independent roles in the etiology of ANV, a number of studies suggest their impact when these patient traits are considered with other clinical characteristics (Table 2). The presence of ANV appears to be associated with more than one variable.

Table 2. Characteristics Affecting Nausea and Vomiting

History of heavy alcohol intake decreases nausea and vomiting

Susceptibility to motion sickness increases nausea and vomiting

Poor previous emetic control increases nausea and vomiting

Younger patients have increased anticipatory nausea and vomiting and increased incidence of dystonic reactions

From Morrow GR. Chemotherapy-related nausea and vomiting: etiology and management. *Cancer.* 1989;39:89–104.

In one of our earlier studies involving 176 cancer patients,[14] significantly more patients who had four or more of the eight characteristics had developed ANV by their fourth chemotherapy treatment. In a follow-up study expanding on these results,[15] we found that patients with three or less of the eight characteristics did not develop ANV. In this study and other explanations, the specificity of the criteria has remained fairly consistent. The eight variables are more valuable in identifying who are not likely to develop anticipatory side effects rather than in identifying patients who will.[5]

The degree to which some of these clinical characteristics are involved in the etiology raises questions about the tremendous individual variation in nausea and vomiting. No study has been able to explain it precisely, but it may be due to some type of interactive etiology. Sweating, feeling warm or hot, and general weakness are likely part of a generalized autonomic reaction to chemotherapy.[3] This reaction may provide for a more intense unconditioned response. Its occurrence prior to nausea and vomiting may lengthen the unconditioned response and shorten the interval between the onset of the unconditioned response and the presentation of the conditioned stimulus.

The potential interrelation among some of the eight clinical characteristics and autonomic changes tends to be supported by a study in five female patients receiving identical cancer chemotherapy and antiemetic drugs.[16] Heart rate, pallor, and skin temperature were assessed during a 1-hour baseline, a 1-hour period of peak nausea, and a 1-hour period of emesis. Temperature and pallor increased linearly from baseline to the periods of nausea and vomiting. Heart rate significantly decreased from baseline to the period of nausea and significantly increased when patients began to vomit. These preliminary findings suggested that nausea may be more related to a rebound of parasympathetic activity than to a slow decrease of sympathetic activity.

Although still preliminary, these results support the emerging view that nausea may involve multiple inputs from the vestibular system, cortical areas of the brain, and other visceral and autonomic signals to a final common pathway.[16] A trend apparent in a number of studies points to a cross-linking between systems. This concept tends to be supported by findings that patients susceptible to motion sickness report greater nausea and emesis with the same chemotherapy drugs than patients who are not prone to motion sickness. Perhaps different pathways predominate for different types of nausea-inducing stimuli.

Behavioral Treatment of ANV

Until more effective antiemetic treatment can control posttreatment nausea and vomiting, ANV will persist because anticipatory side effects largely reflect the failure of antiemetic management in the posttreatment setting.

Paradoxically, as more effective antiemetics are developed, increasingly aggressive chemotherapy protocols will be used, which will once again limit the effectiveness of antiemetic regimens.

Because antiemetic medications are ineffective in controlling anticipatory symptoms, attention has focused on behavioral strategies.

Three principal behavioral interventions have been studied for their potential benefit in controlling ANV: *hypnosis, progressive relaxation training,* and *systematic desensitization.*

Hypnosis

Hypnosis is probably more useful in children than in adults. Adults tend to be more skeptical of its potential; the early history of hypnosis and its connotation as a sideshow or gimmick still raise questions about its legitimacy as a therapeutic tool. In children, however, case studies suggest that the technique may effectively control some undesirable symptoms.

LaBaw et al,[17] reported case studies of 27 children and adolescents treated with nonstandardized self-hypnosis over 2 years. Using progressive body relaxation as induction, investigators employed imagery of idyllic scenes and achieved variable success. Generally, the technique improved sleep, increased caloric intake and retention, increased fluid intake, and helped patients tolerate therapeutic procedures.

Mixed results from controlled studies, however, raise questions about the duration of the effectiveness of hypnosis and whether its apparent benefits may be explained by other factors. In a study of six patients,[18] symptoms that apparently had been controlled by hypnosis reappeared after an unavoidable interruption of hypnotherapy in some patients. Another study reported a significant reduction in the intensity and severity of nausea and vomiting and an increase in oral intake over two chemotherapy cycles in hypnotized patients compared with controls, but the authors question whether such benefits could be attributable to the extra attention the children received from the therapist.

Progressive Relaxation Training

With *progressive relaxation training* (PRT), patients learn to relax by actively tensing and relaxing muscle groups in a progressive manner. Typically, an individual is taught deep muscle relaxation by a therapist; a training audiotape is made, and the patient then practices PRT at home. Results from case studies indicate that PRT helps reduce side effects such as postchemotherapy nausea and vomiting, as well as depression and anxiety. Although not confirmed, PRT may help manage or prevent ANV either directly or by controlling of postchemotherapy nausea and vomiting.

Two studies in cancer patients tend to support the value of PRT in this setting. In the first, Lyles et al[19] studied 50 anxious and depressed patients who were also nauseated and vomiting. Those patients who received PRT with guided imagery had a reduction in these side effects, both during and following their chemotherapy sessions, compared with patients in two control groups (therapist attention or no treatment). In the other study involving 43 cancer patients, 67% of those undergoing PRT had increases in postchemotherapy nausea and vomiting, compared to 85% of patients in two control groups.[20]

Timing may be an important factor in the effectiveness of PRT. In the first reported study involving PRT as a preventive strategy, Burish et al[21] assessed its ability to prevent or ameliorate side effects of chemotherapy. The 32 cancer patients about to start chemotherapy were randomly assigned to either a PRT group or an untreated control group. Patients who had PRT sessions prior to initiation of chemotherapy and during the first five treatments reported less nausea, vomiting, and lower physiologic arousal during and following chemotherapy. By the fifth session, only 10% of PRT patients experienced nausea following chemotherapy, compared with 54% of controls.[21]

Overall, the data suggest that PRT is a useful tool in reducing side effects during and after cancer chemotherapy. The optimal timing of PRT appears to be prior to the first chemotherapy session, when it has potential to block the conditioning process.

Systematic Desensitization

With *systematic desensitization*, situations likely to elicit ANV are counter-conditioned by conditioning patients to a response that is incompatible with nausea and vomiting.[2] For example, patients are taught a response (such as relaxation) that is incompatible with the maladaptive response (ANV) to particular stimuli.[1] While deeply relaxed, patients image scenes from a hierarchy of events related to ANV (such as the sequence of driving to the cancer center and seeing the treatment nurse). Soon patients have learned to associate treatment stimuli with relaxation rather than with nausea and vomiting.

In a case study of 60 patients with ANV, we found that only those patients in the systematic desensitization group showed a significant reduction in the frequency, severity, and duration of ANV compared with patients in two control groups (Rogerian client-centered therapy and no treatment).[22] The efficacy of systematic desensitization appeared unrelated to antiemetic medications used by the patients, their expectation of improvement, or nonspecific effects of therapy.

As is the case with PRT, the timing of systematic desensitization appears to influence its potential for success. Dobkin[23] examined the effect of systematic desensitization before the second chemotherapy session in 40 patients. Those undergoing systematic desensitization had less frequent, less severe, and shorter episodes of postchemotherapy nausea and vomiting than control patients. This study suggested that the technique may be able to reduce the development of conditioned side effects resulting from chemotherapy.

Systematic desensitization can be taught to patients in about 20 minutes. Properly trained nurses and oncologists can use the technique with about the same effectiveness as trained behavioral consultants.[24] Our recent study in 72 cancer patients failed to find significant differences in effectiveness when systematic desensitization was delivered by medical personnel or by clinical psychologists.[24] Nurses and oncologists were able to use systematic desensitization as successfully, and in some cases more effectively, as clinical psychologists. Possibly because the patients saw the oncology staff for longer periods and more often than they saw the psychology experimenters, subsequent chemotherapy sessions in the clinic may have reinforced the potential of behavioral relaxation. This theory, however, is still speculative and needs supporting data from controlled trials. The finding that desensitization by oncologists and nurses was more effective in reducing the incidence of posttreatment vomiting than desensitization by psychologists may reflect the theory that posttreatment chemotherapy side effects are learned. Clinic personnel ordinarily are conditioned stimuli that elicit posttreatment side effects. But by applying systematic desensitization, the staff become actively involved as agents of change, and their presence no longer elicits side effects but rather reduces them. Regardless of the mechanisms involved, these results may encourage medical personnel to learn and successfully use systematic desensitization and other behavioral interventions to prevent the development of ANV and posttreatment nausea and vomiting.

Conclusion

New models delineating the etiology of ANV have more clearly explained mechanisms potentially responsible for the development of this complication. It appears that ANV is learned and that classical learning theory can account for the high prevalence of side effects in patients undergoing chemotherapy. That is, ANV is rooted in a sequence of classically conditioned responses that develop after patients have undergone a series of chemotherapy treatments. The severity of posttreatment nausea and vomiting is significantly associated with the development of ANV. However, the association of other factors, including anxiety and various clinical characteristics, suggests that ANV may involve a more complex etiology that is not based solely on learning.

Eight clinical characteristics can help predict the occurrence of ANV: (1) nausea or vomiting after the last chemotherapy session; (2) posttreatment nausea moderate, severe, or intolerable; (3) posttreatment vomiting moderate, severe, or intolerable; (4) age less than 50 years; (5) susceptibility to motion sickness; (6) generalized weakness after the last session; (7) sweating after the last chemotherapy session; (8) feeling warm or hot after the last chemotherapy session.

Because antiemetic medications are ineffective in ANV, management has focused on the use of behavioral interventions. Progressive relaxation training and systematic desensitization have produced the most benefit and can be as effectively used by nurses and oncologists as by clinical psychologists.

References

1. Morrow GR, Burish TG, Bellg A. Treatment of anticipatory nausea and vomiting. In: Rubio ED, Martin M, eds. *Antiemetic Therapy: Current Status and Future Prospects.* Madrid, Spain: Creationes Elba, SA; 1992:181–189.

2. Morrow GR. Chemotherapy-related nausea and vomiting: etiology and management. *Cancer.* 1989;39:89–104.

3. Morrow GR, Lindke JL, Black PM. Predicting development of anticipatory nausea in cancer patients: prospective examination of eight clinical characteristics. *J Pain Symptom Manag.* 1991;6:215–223.

4. Morrow GR, Dobkin PL. Anticipatory nausea and vomiting.in cancer patients undergoing chemotherapy treatment: prevalence, etiology, and behavioral interventions. *Clin Psych Rev.* 1988;8:517–556.

5. Morrow GR, Lindke JL, Black PM. Anticipatory nausea development in cancer patients: replication and extension of a learning model. *Br J Psychol.* 1991;82:61–69.

6. Redd WH, Andrykowski MA. Behavioral intervention in cancer treatment: controlling aversion reactions to chemotherapy. *J Consult Clin Psych.* 1982;50:1018–1029.

7. Nicholas DR. Prevalence of anticipatory nausea and emesis in cancer chemotherapy patients. *J Behav Med.* 1982;5:461–462.

8. Dobkin P, Zeichner A, Dickson-Parnell B. Concomitants of anticipatory nausea and emesis in cancer chemotherapy. *Psych Rep.* 1985;56:671–676.

9. Robertson RG, Garcia J. X-rays and learned taste aversions: historical and psychological ramifications. In: Burish TG, Levy SM, Myerowitz BE, eds. *Cancer, Nutrition, and Eating Behavior: A Biobehavioral Perspective.* Hillsdale, NJ: Erlbaum; 1985:11–41.

10. Andrykowski MA, Redd WH, Hatfield AK. Development of anticipatory nausea: a prospective analysis. *J Consult Clin Psych.* 1985;53:447–454.

11. Morrow GR. Behaviorial factors influencing the development and expression of chemotherapy induced side effects. *Brit J Cancer.* 1992;66:S54–S61.

12. Love RR, Nerenz DR, Leventhal H. Anticipatory nausea with cancer chemotherapy: development through two mechanisms. Proceedings of the annual meeting of the American Society of Clinical Oncology. 1982;2:242.

13. Andrykowski MA. Do infusion-related tastes and odors facilitate the development of anticipatory nausea? A failure to support hypothesis. *Health Psych.* 1987;6:329–341.

14. Morrow GR. Clinical characteristics associated with the development of anticipatory nausea and vomiting in cancer patients undergoing chemotherapy treatment. *J Clin Oncol.* 1984;2:1170–1178.

15. Morrow GR, Waight J, Black PM. Anticipatory nausea development in cancer patients: replication and extension of a learning model. *Br J Psycol.* 1991;82:61–72.

16. Morrow GR, Angel C, Dubeshter B. Autonomic changes during cancer chemotherapy induced nausea and emesis. *Brit J Cancer.* 1992;66:S42–S45.

17. LaBaw W, Holton C, Tewell K, Eccles D. The use of self-hypnosis by children with cancer. *Am J Clin Hypnosis.* 1975;17:233–238.

18. Redd WH, Anderson GU, Minigawa RY. Hypnotic control of anticipatory emesis in cancer patients receiving chemotherapy. *J Consult Clin Psychol.* 1982;50:14–22.

19. Lyles JN, Burish TG, Krozely MG, et al. Efficacy of relaxation training and guided imagery in reducing the aversiveness of cancer chemotherapy. *J Consult Clin Psychol.* 1982;50:509–517.

20. Cotanch PH. Muscle relaxation versus "attention-placebo" in decreasing the aversiveness of chemotherapy. Unpublished manuscript. Duke University; 1983.

21. Burish TG, Carey MP, Krozely MG, et al. Conditioned side effects induced by cancer chemotherapy: prevention through behavioral treatment. *J Consult Clin Psychol.* 1987;55:1–9.

22. Morrow GR, Morrell C. Behavioral treatment for the anticipatory nausea and vomiting induced by cancer chemotherapy. *N Engl J Med.* 1982;307:1476–1483.

23. Dobkin P. The use of systematic desensitization, a behavioral intervention, in the reduction of aversive chemotherapy side effects in cancer patients. Unpublished doctoral dissertation. University of Georgia, Athens; 1987.

24. Morrow GR, Asbury R, Caruso L, et al. Comparing the effectiveness of behavioral treatment for chemotherapy induced nausea/vomiting when administered by oncologists, oncology nurses or clinical psychologists. *Health Psychology.* 1992;11:250–256.

Diagnosis and Management of Vertigo

Robert W. Baloh, MD

Nausea and vomiting are among the autonomic symptoms commonly associated with vertigo. But vertigo is not the most common type of dizziness—in our experience, less than half of patients complaining of dizziness actually have vertigo.[1] Dizziness may be due to any number of changes in the brain centers that integrate visual, proprioceptive, and vestibular signals. Nausea and vomiting and other autonomic symptoms such as sweating and pallor are uncommon with types of dizziness other than vertigo. These autonomic symptoms are important because of their association with vestibular lesions.

Extremely frightening to the patient and often characterized by abrupt onset, vertigo is an illusion of movement, usually rotation, although patients occasionally describe a sensation of linear displacement or tilt. An imbalance anywhere in the peripheral and central vestibular pathways can lead to an illusion of movement. The same sensation can result from lesions in such diverse locations as the inner ear, the deep paravertebral stretch receptors of the neck, the visual-vestibular interaction centers in the brain stem and cerebellum, and the subjective sensation pathways of the thalamus and cortex.[2]

Compared with nonvestibular dizziness, vertigo tends to be characterized by an episodic rather than a continuous pattern (Table 1). After an abrupt onset, the intensity of vertigo decreases as the inciting factor dissipates or as compensation occurs.[1] Patients with vestibular disorders are not likely to experience continuous dizziness, because even with a complete unilateral loss of vestibular function, vertigo gradually resolves as central compensation occurs.

Vertigo is usually aggravated by head movements rather than by visual targets. Rapid head movements provoke vertigo because they accentuate imbalances within the vestibular system.

Vertigo should be differentiated from other common causes of dizziness: (1) presyncopal lightheadedness caused by diffuse cerebral ischemia;

Table 1. Distinguishing between Vestibular and Nonvestibular Types of Dizziness

	Vestibular	Nonvestibular
Common descriptive terms	Spinning (environment moves), merry-go-round, drunkeness, tilting, motion sickness, off-balance	Lightheaded, floating, dissociated from body, swimming, giddy, spinning inside (environment stationary)
Course	Episodic	Constant
Common participating factors	Head movements, position change	Stress, hyperventilation, cardiac arrhythmia situations
Common associated symptoms	Nausea, vomiting, unsteadiness, tinnitus, hearing loss, impaired vision, oscillopsia	Perspiration, palor, paresthesias, palpitations, syncope, difficulty concentrating, tension headache

From Baloh RW, Honrubia V. Clinical Neurophysiology of the Vestibular System. Philadelphia: F.A. Davis Company, 1990.

(2) psychophysiologic dizziness associated with impaired central integration of sensory signals; (3) dysequilibrium associated with loss of vestibulospinal, proprioceptive, cerebellar, or motor function; (4) ocular dizziness due to visual-vestibular mismatch in patients with impaired vision; (5) multisensory dizziness caused by partial loss of multiple sensory system function; and (6) physiologic dizziness, due to conflict from an unusual combination of sensory signals.

Regardless of the cause of dizziness, the physician needs to provide support and reassurance. If the patient's fear and anxiety can be alleviated, the symptom is less distressing.[3] Patients often think that vertigo indicates a brain tumor or another life-threatening neurologic disorder.

Important distinctions can help differentiate peripheral (end-organ and nerve) and central causes of vertigo. In vertigo associated with a peripheral cause, nausea and vomiting are severe; imbalance is mild; hearing loss is common; oscillopsia is mild; neurologic symptoms are rare; and compensation is rapid (Table 2). Typically, but not always, autonomic symptoms are more pronounced when the vertigo has a peripheral origin. Well-documented lesions within the vestibular pathways sometimes produce only a nonspecific sensation of disorientation, without a clearly defined illusion of movement.[1] Normal subjects undergoing caloric stimulation—a

Table 2. Differentiation between Peripheral (End-Organ and Nerve) and Central Causes of Vertigo

	Nausea and Vomiting	Imbalance	Hearing Loss	Oscillopsia	Neurologic Symptoms	Compensation
Peripheral	Severe	Mild	Common	Mild	Rare	Rapid
Central	Moderate	Severe	Rare	Severe	Common	Slow

From Baloh RW, Honrubia V. *Clinical Neurophysiology of the Vestibular System*. Philadelphia: F.A. Davis Company; 1990.

physiologic imbalance in the vestibular system—occasionally report a floating sensation or even giddiness. This example illustrates why subjective criteria alone cannot be used to classify dizziness.

Vestibular Disorders

Once a vestibular disorder is suspected, the evaluation can focus on differentiating between common disorders or syndromes that may be the cause of vertigo.

Benign Positional Vertigo

Benign positional vertigo is not a disease but rather a syndrome that can be the sequela of several different inner ear diseases. In about half of these cases, no cause can be found.[4,5] Benign positional vertigo is the most commonly identified form of vertigo, and it can be treated with relative ease.

The syndrome is characterized by brief episodes of vertigo (<30 seconds) typically precipitated by change in position. It is most common when turning over in bed, getting in and out of bed, bending over and straightening up, and extending the neck to look up. So-called "top-shelf vertigo," vertigo that occurs while reaching for something on a high shelf, is nearly always due to benign positional vertigo. Diagnosis rests on finding a characteristic fatigable paroxysmal positional nystagmus after the patient rapidly changes from the sitting to the head-hanging position (the Hallpike maneuver). Patients can be reassured that episodes of benign positional vertigo remit spontaneously and do not merit an extensive work-up.

Studies of the temporal bone in patients with benign positional vertigo identified basophilic deposits on the cupula of the posterior semicircular canal.[6] These deposits were prominent only on the side that was lower when paroxysmal positional nystagmus and vertigo were induced. The

29

deposits were probably otoconia released from a degenerating utricular macula. The otoconia settled on the cupula of the posterior canal (situated directly under the utricular macule) making it more sensitive to changes in the direction of gravity.

The change from a sitting to a head-hanging position causes the posterior canal to move from an inferior to a superior position. A utriculofugal displacement of the cupula occurs, triggering a burst of nystagmus. Consistent with this theory, the burst of paroxysmal positional nystagmus is in the plane of the posterior canal of the lower ear, with the fast component directed upward. This would be predicted from ampullofugal stimulation of the posterior canal.[7,8]

The clinical course of the syndrome is suggested by a review of 240 cases of benign positional vertigo.[9] The episode of dizziness never lasted more than 1 minute. However, in many patients a flurry of episodes preceded nausea and more prolonged, nonspecific dizziness (lightheadedness, swimming sensation) that lasted for hours to days. Typically, bouts of benign positional vertigo were intermixed with variable periods of remission. The onset of these episodes occurred at a mean age of 54 years, and one third of patients reported that the syndrome had been present for more than 10 years. No cause could be identified in about half the cases. Posttraumatic and postviral neurolabyrinthitis were the most common diagnoses in the remainder of the patients. Positional vertigo presented within 3 days of head trauma in patients with posttraumatic neurolabyrinthitis. Patients with viral neurolabyrinthitis reported a prior episode of acute vertigo that gradually resolved within 2 weeks.

Despite the benign nature of the syndrome, its frequently prolonged clinical course is worrisome to patients. A simple explanation of the disorder and reassurance about its favorable prognosis can help relieve anxiety, but patients should also be warned about the likelihood of a recurrence. Treatment focuses on positional exercises, medications, and, rarely, surgery in prolonged cases.

Positional exercises can accelerate remissions in most cases of benign positional vertigo.[10] The patient sits on the edge of a bed and then rapidly assumes the lateral position to induce positional vertigo (Fig 1). After the vertigo subsides, the patient returns to the upright position. These positional changes are repeated three times a day, until the vertigo tends to subside. Patients whose vertigo shows prominent fatigue on the standard diagnostic positional test benefit most from these exercises.[1] Effectiveness of the positional exercises may be due to either dislodgement of the calcium carbonate material from the cupula of the posterior semicircular canal[10] or central adaptation.

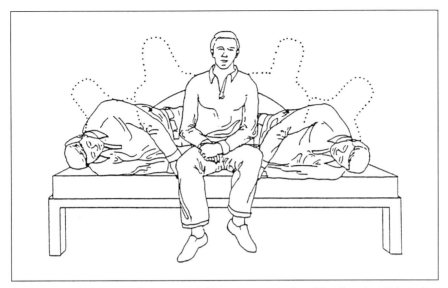

Fig 1. Positioning exercises for treatment of benign paroxysmal positional vertigo. (Adapted from Brandt T, Daroff RB. Physical therapy for benign paroxysmal positional vertigo. *Arch Otolaryngol.* 1980;106:484.)

The short duration of positional vertigo tends to complicate therapy. Heavy sedation would be required throughout the day to completely suppress the brief episodes. Symptomatic treatment with an antivertigo medication such as meclizine or promethazine (25 mg each) is often effective for acute exacerbations while the patient is performing positional exercises. Although they suppress the nausea and nonspecific dizziness between acute episodes, these agents only minimally affect the abrupt episodes.

Patients refractory to conventional therapy may be candidates for singular neurectomy, a surgical procedure in which the ampullary nerve is sectioned from the posterior semicircular canal crista. The procedure is effective in more than 90% of patients, but it causes sensorineural hearing loss in 8%. An alternative procedure, transection of the vestibular nerve through the middle cranial fossa, is associated with greater risks than singular neurectomy.[1] A new procedure for surgically blocking the posterior semicircular canal is now being evaluated.

Meniere's Syndrome

The hallmark symptoms of Meniere's syndrome include fullness and pressure along with impaired hearing in one ear. The course of the disease varies in its early stages, but the diagnosis hinges on the presence of fluctuating hearing loss and vertigo. At first, intensifying rapidly within minutes, vertigo slowly subsides over several hours, but the patient usually is left with a sense of unsteadiness and dizziness for days after the acute vertiginous episode. Tinnitus, usually described as a roar, may persist between episodes; it usually intensifies immediately before or after the acute episode.[1] After vomiting, the patient prefers to lie in bed without eating until the acute symptoms pass. This pattern occurs irregularly for years, interrupted by periods of remission. A severe and permanent hearing loss eventually sets in, and the episodes disappear.

The main pathologic finding in patients with Meniere's syndrome is distension of the endolymphatic system.[11,12] The membranous labyrinth progressively dilates until the sacular wall makes contact with the footplate of the stapes and the cochlear duct occupies the entire vestibular scala. The cochlear and vestibular end-organs and nerves show minimal pathologic changes. Herniations and ruptures of the membranous labyrinth are common, the latter frequently involving Reissner's membrane and the walls of the sacculus, utriculus, and ampullae. Occasionally, rupture is followed by complete collapse of the membranous labyrinth.

The underlying mechanism for the fluctuating symptoms and signs of the syndrome is still unclear. The episodes of hearing loss and vertigo may be caused by ruptures in the membrane, which separate endolymph from perilymph and produce a sudden rise in potassium levels in the latter.[13] As potassium slowly clears over several hours, symptoms and signs subside. An alternative explanation implicates mechanical deformation of the end-organ that is reversible as the endolymphatic pressure decreases. The infrequent but dramatic and sudden falling attacks seen in patients with Meniere's syndrome are most likely due to a sudden deformation or displacement of one of the vestibular sense organs.[14]

The diagnosis of Meniere's syndrome is best secured by documentation of fluctuating hearing levels. The following signs are helpful in confirming the diagnosis:

- A shift of more than 10 dB occurs at two different frequencies.
- In early stages, the sensorineural hearing loss is usually greater at lower frequencies.
- Electronystagmography (ENG) may reveal peripheral spontaneous nystagmus and either vestibular paresis or directional preponderance on caloric testing.
- During an acute attack, the nystagmus may be directed toward the involved ear, suggesting an excitatory rather than a destructive effect.
- Computerized x-rays of the temporal bones in patients with idiopathic Meniere's syndrome often show narrowing of the endolymphatic duct or decreased pneumatization of the temporal bone.[15]

The cornerstones of therapy in Meniere's syndrome are symptomatic treatment of acute episodes and long-term prophylaxis with salt restriction and diuretics.[16,17] Acute vertigo, nausea, and vomiting usually respond to promethazine (25 mg to 50 mg). It should be taken as early as possible, preferably during the prodrome if symptoms are apparent. Occasionally, an antiemetic agent such as prochlorperazine is of benefit. Although it is unclear precisely why salt restriction is effective, the results can be dramatic. Patients with debilitating symptoms have shown prolonged remissions that last years when they maintain a low-salt diet. Yet salt restriction may have little or no effect in other patients, reflecting the multifactorial pathogenesis of the syndrome and the need for empiric treatment. We recommend salt restriction of 1 gm per day for a minimum of 2 to 3 months. If this is effective, then the level of salt intake can be gradually increased while symptoms and signs are carefully monitored. Fluid and food intake should be distributed regularly throughout the day, and binges (particularly of food with high sugar and/or salt content) should be avoided. Adjunctive therapy with diuretics may provide additional benefit in some patients, but it cannot substitute for a low-salt diet.

Patients who are candidates for surgery may be referred for either endolymphatic shunts or destructive procedures. Although shunts are logical because of the presumed pathophysiology of Meniere's syndrome, their efficacy is limited by several factors. The aim of the most popular shunt is to drain the endolymphatic sac to the mastoid cavity, but the success of this procedure may be hindered by blockage of the endolymphatic pathways proximal to the endolymphatic sac. Another potential problem, according to Schuknecht,[18] is that a drain device implanted in the endolymphatic sac will almost certainly become rapidly encapsulated in fibrous tissue. Consequently, the use of this technique is controversial.

The other surgical approach, ablation, is based on the theory that the nervous system can compensate for complete loss of vestibular function better than it can compensate for a fluctuating, partial loss. Ablation is most effective in patients with unilateral involvement and no functional hearing on the damaged side. Vestibular nerve section is recommended for patients with functional residual hearing. Vertigo is expected early after surgery, but most patients can resume normal activity within 1 to 3 months if they follow a structured program of vestibular exercises. Destructive surgical procedures generally should be avoided in elderly patients, who do not adjust well to vestibular imbalance.

Viral Neurolabyrinthitis

The clinical features of viral neurolabyrinthitis can include sudden deafness (usually unilateral), acute vertigo (with associated autonomic symptoms), or some combination of auditory and vestibular symptoms. Deafness due to viral infection generally develops over several hours and may extend over several days,[19] although more than half of such patients recover whether or not they are treated. The characteristic features of vestibular neurolabyrinthitis are vertigo, nausea, and vomiting developing over several hours, usually peaking within 24 hours and resolving over several weeks. During the first day, the patient has severe truncal unsteadiness and imbalance and difficulty focusing because of spontaneous nystagmus.

Although most patients recover completely within 3 months, some patients, especially the elderly, have residual problems, including intractable dizziness, for years. Vertigo recurs at least once in 20% to 30% of patients, although the repeat episode is usually less severe. The reoccurrence may signify reactivation of a latent virus, because it is often associated with systemic viral illness.

The key to the diagnosis lies in the characteristic clinical profile along with evidence of peripheral auditory and/or vestibular dysfunction in the absence of neurologic symptoms and signs. Partial hearing loss is most apparent in the high frequencies and indicates damage in the basilar turn of the cochlea. Brain stem evoked response studies are usually normal, consistent with a cochlear site of pathology.

Viral neurolabyrinthitis should be differentiated from bacterial and syphilitic illnesses, as well as from acute labyrinthine ischemia and perilymph fistula. Bacterial labyrinthitis is relatively easy to recognize because of its frequent association with acute and chronic otomastoiditis, and it can be verified by examination of the ear and by computed tomography of the temporal bone. Syphilitic labyrinthitis characteristically leads to recurrent vertigo and hearing loss and progresses to severe bilateral dysfunction over a period of months; in contrast, unilateral vestibular loss is seen with viral labyrinthitis. The onset of symptoms is an important factor in differentiating infarction of the labyrinth; the sudden, profound loss of auditory and vestibular function contrasts sharply with the gradual onset of symptoms in viral labyrinthitis. Onset of symptoms—hearing loss, vertigo, or a combination of auditory and vestibular symptoms—is also abrupt with perilymph fistula. A precipitating event such as head trauma, barotrauma, or sudden strain during lifting, coughing, or sneezing is often associated with these symptoms.

Patients with isolated episodes of auditory and/or vestibular loss should be managed presumptively with symptomatic treatment, unless convincing evidence points to vascular or nonviral infection. Vestibular exercises should be started immediately after the acute nausea and vomiting subside, and they should be continued until dizziness and imbalance are minimal.[3]

The use of drug therapy in patients presumed to have viral labyrinthitis is less clear because the pathophysiology is often uncertain. Steroids have been recommended for their anti-inflammatory benefits, but the risk/benefit ratio of steriods in this setting has not been adequately studied. Antiviral agents such as cytosine arabinase and acyclovir have been effective in treating systemic viral illnesses in children, but it is uncertain whether they alter the hearing loss associated with disorders such as cytomegalovirus and rubella. Studies are needed to determine whether antiviral agents can be effective in adults with presumed viral neurolabyrinthitis.

Vascular Disorders

Vertebrobasilar Insufficiency

A common cause of vertigo in patients older than 65 years, vertebrobasilar insufficiency (VBI) usually is caused by atherosclerosis of the subclavian, vertebral, and basilar arteries. Vertigo is the initial symptom in nearly half the patients with VBI.[20] The vertigo is abrupt in onset and frequently is associated with nausea and vomiting. Invariably, the vertigo also is associated with symptoms resulting from ischemia in the territory supplied by the posterior circulation. Vertigo may be an isolated initial symptom of VBI, or, it may occur in isolation and also intermixed with more typical episodes of VBI.[21] Another disorder should be suspected if episodes of vertigo recur for more than 6 months without other symptoms.

Diagnostic studies should focus on finding a combination of symptoms that typically occur in VBI episodes, which last only minutes. In addition to vertigo, these symptoms include visual loss or hallucinations, drop attacks or weakness, visceral sensations, visual field defects, diplopia, and headaches. Patients commonly have a history of myocardial infarction or occlusive peripheral vascular disease related to atherosclerosis. When evaluations are performed between episodes of vertigo, patients appear normal neurologically, but they may show residual signs of brain stem and/or cerebellar infarction.

Both peripheral and central signs can occur on ENG testing, the most common being unilateral vestibular paresis with caloric stimulation, which occurs in about 25% of patients[21]; it is probably caused by ischemic damage to the vestibular labyrinth. Computed tomography and magnetic resonance scans are likely to be normal. Angiography often is not correlated with clinical symptoms and signs, and is unlikely to serve as a basis for surgery.

Management.   Most patients with VBI do not develop infarction. At greatest risk are patients who present with episodes of quadriparesis, perioral numbness, bilateral blindness, or loss of consciousness. These symptoms may foreshadow basilar artery thrombosis, and their presence calls for aggressive investigation.

Modification of atherosclerotic risk factors (diabetes, hypertension, hyperlipidemia) and antiplatelet therapy (aspirin, 330 mg/day) are important in management of patients with VBI. Anticoagulation is reserved for patients with frequent incapacitating episodes and for patients with signs and symptoms suggesting a stroke in evolution, particularly basilar artery thrombosis.

Intravenous heparin, beginning with a bolus of 5000 units followed by a continuous infusion of 1000 units per hour, is recommended. The dose is titrated to keep the partial thromboplastin time at approximately 2.5 times the control value.[1] After 3 to 4 days, warfarin is begun at an oral dose of 15 mg, adjusted until the prothrombin time is approximately twice the control value. When heparin is discontinued at this point, some patients will experience a recurrence of symptoms, necessitating reinstitution of the drug and then a gradual tapering.

Surgery has not been successful in the vertebrobasilar system. Specific indications for surgery need further definition. Controlled studies using modern angiographic and surgical techniques are needed to assess the risk/benefit ratio.

Migraine

The periodic headaches of migraine are often associated with dizziness and vertigo. Nearly always familial, migraine reportedly affects nearly 25% of women and 15% of men,[22] usually before age 40. Vertigo can occur with the headaches or in separate episodes, and it can predate the onset of headache. The extent to which vertigo is associated with migraine is apparent in a study comparing the incidence of nonspecific dizziness (a giddy sensation) and vertigo in 200 patients with migraine and 116 patients with tension headache.[23] The incidence of nonspecific dizziness was similar in the migraine and tension headache groups (28% and 22% respectively), but the migraine patients reported a much higher incidence of vertigo than the tension headache patients (27% vs. 8%). The severity of vertigo per se prompted 10 patients with migraine to seek help.

Types of Migraine
Depending on the pattern of symptoms, migraines are grouped into four categories: (1) classic migraine, (2) common migraine, (3) posterior fossa migraine, and (4) migraine equivalents.

The following characteristics describe classic migraine:

- The headache begins with an aura and continues with a severe, throbbing, usually unilateral headache.
- Aura symptoms slowly progress over several minutes, last 15 to 60 minutes, and then gradually abate. However, the onset is abrupt in 25% of patients.
- The headache begins as the aura diminishes, usually peaking in about an hour and gradually subsiding over the next 4 to 8 hours.
- Nausea and vomiting typically accompany the onset of head pain.

The migraine aura consists of transient neurologic dysfunction, usually visual disturbances, and sometimes prominent vertigo or somatosensory symptoms. Visual phenomena include blindness, hemianopia or quadrantanopia, tunnel vision, altitudinal defects, monocular blindness, and scotoma. Patients also report seeing stars, sparkling lights, unformed flashes of light, geometric patterns, or a jagged, sparkling zigzag.

In contrast to the classic migraine, the aura phenomena are absent in common migraine. The headache, unilateral or bilateral, slowly intensifies and may last for several days. It is often accompanied by nausea, vomiting, diarrhea, chills, and prostration. Nonspecific dizziness is a common complaint, and patients frequently report visual blurring and a sense of unsteadiness.

Posterior fossa migraine is differentiated by an aura consisting of posterior fossa symptoms, such as vertigo, ataxia, dysarthria, and tinnitus, along with visual phenomena consistent with ischemia in the distribution of the posterior cerebral arteries. The vertigo usually has an abrupt onset and lasts 5 to 60 minutes.[24] Posterior fossa migraine should be suspected in any patient presenting with transient vertigo and other posterior fossa symptoms.

Episodic disorders in which headache is not always present have been called migraine equivalents. Presenting features may include repeated or cyclic periods of vertigo, vomiting, attacks of abdominal pain, or ophthalmoplegia. These symptoms may begin in adulthood and may be accompanied by attacks of paresthesia, aphasia, dysarthria, paresis, or diplopia, with or without the visual manifestations of migraine. A migraine syndrome is diagnosed despite the absence of associated headaches.

Diagnosis and Management

The following criteria have been suggested for diagnosing migraine headaches[25]: recurrent headaches separated by symptom-free intervals; any three of the following six symptoms: abdominal pain, nausea, or vomiting during the headache; hemicrania; a throbbing or pulsate quality to the

Table 3. Dosage and Effects of Commonly Used Antivertiginous Medications

Class	Drug	Dosage
Anticholinergic	Scopolamine	0.6 mg orally q4–6h or 0.5 mg transdermally q3d
Monoaminergic	Amphetamine	5 or 10 mg orally q4–6h
	Ephedrine	25 mg orally q4–6h
Antihistamine	Meclizine (Antivert)	25 mg orally q4–6h
	Dimenhydrinate (Dramamine)	50 mg orally or intramuscularly q4–6h or 100-mg suppository q8h
	Promethazine (Phenergan)	25 or 50 mg orally, intramuscularly, or as suppository q4–6h
Phenothiazine	Prochlorperazine (Compazine)	5 or 10 mg orally or intramuscularly q6h or 25 mg suppository q12h
Benzodiazepine	Diazepam (Valium)	5 or 10 mg orally, intramuscularly, or intravenously q4-6h

pain; complete relief after a brief period of rest; an aura (visual, sensory, or motor); and a history of migraine headaches in one or more members of the immediate family.

Symptomatic treatment of migraine emphasizes analgesics, antiemetics, antivertigo drugs, sedatives, and vasoconstrictors. Because the decrease in gastric motility during a migraine attack may interfere with drug absorption and contribute to nausea and vomiting, metoclopramide may be of benefit. Combination agents for symptomatic relief that contain sedatives are effective partially because they enhance sleep.

Sedation	Antiemetic Actions	Dryness of Mucous Membranes	Extrapyramidal Symptoms
+	+	+ + +	−
−	+	+	+
−	+	+	−
+	+	+	−
+	+	+	−
+ +	+ +	+	−
+	+ + +	+	+ + +
+ + +	+	−	−

From Baloh RW, Honrubia V. *Clinical Neurophysiology of the Vestibular System.* Philadelphia: F.A. Davis Company; 1990.

Ergotamine, probably the most effective drug for treatment of migraine, acts as a vasoconstrictor when vascular resistance is low but induces vasodilation when resistance is increased. However, if use of ergotamine is associated with severe nausea and vomiting despite the administration of metoclopramide, other agents may need to be considered. Administration of ergotamine is recommended as soon as possible after the onset of symptoms.

Antivertigo and antiemetic medications are advised when vertigo and nausea are the prominent features (Table 3). Promethazine is often the drug of choice. When symptomatic treatment fails, prophylactic therapy is useful, preferably propranolol, the only FDA-approved drug for prophylactic use in migraine. Up to 70% of propranolol-treated patients respond.[26,27] Adults usually require 120 to 360 mg per day, and the drug should be continued for at least 2 to 3 months. Other drugs showing promise in the treatment of migraine include amitriptyline (especially when episodes are triggered by tension or closely associated with tension headache) and calcium channel blockers. It is unknown, whether calcium channel blockers are as effective as propranolol because long-term data are unavailable. Any patient with migraine, episodes of vertigo, and a strong family history should undergo a trial of migraine prophylaxis.

Symptomatic Treatment of Vertigo

Ideally, if the underlying disorder is identified, treatment can be specific. But in most cases, symptomatic treatment is combined with specific therapy or may be the only therapy available. Symptomatic treatment includes antivertigo medications and vestibular exercises.

The use of antivertigo drugs is based on empirical grounds. It is difficult to predict in which patients they will be effective. The mechanism of action of these drugs is unclear, although most either decrease the efficacy of transmission from primary to secondary vestibular neurons or decrease the overall excitability of neurons in the vestibular nucleus. Drug selection should take into consideration the known effects of each agent and the severity and duration of symptoms (Table 3). For example, in patients with episodes of severe vertigo, in whom sedation is desirable, promethazine and diazepam are useful. Sedation is also desirable in patients with chronic and recurrent vertigo, for whom meclizine, dimenhydrinate, and scopolamine may be indicated. In cases of severe nausea and vomiting, the antiemetic prochlorperazine can be combined with an antivertigo medication. Among the antihistamines, promethazine's strong sedating effects need to be considered. The combination of promethazine and the sympathomimetic ephedrine is less sedating and more effective in relieving associated autonomic symptoms.

Exercise as soon as possible after a labyrinthine injury or ablation has long been considered beneficial. Vestibular exercises are designed to gradually retrain the eye and body musculature to use vision and proprioceptive signals to compensate for lost vestibular signals. Patients should perform eye and head movements in bed as soon as possible after acute vertigo, nausea, and vomiting have subsided, and they should begin the remaining exercises as they recover. Three 5-minute exercise sessions per day are recommended.

One of the goals of these exercises is to identify head positions and movements that cause dizziness within tolerable limits; the more frequently dizziness is induced, the more quickly a patient is likely to compensate.

Group exercise should be encouraged, because patients tend to support each other and can note the progress made by others over the long term. Each patient should receive instructions on how to exercise, and should be given written guidelines outlining the regimen. During the 1 to 3 months when exercises are continued, patients should be encouraged to resume normal activity.

References

1. Baloh RW, Honrubia V. The history in the dizzy patient: treatment options. In: *Clinical Neurophysiology of the Vestibular System*. Philadelphia: F.A. Davis; 1990:91–111.
2. Baloh RW. The dizzy patient. In: Hachinski V, ed. *Challenges in Neurology*. Philadelphia: F.A. Davis; 1992:15–27.
3. Baloh RW. The dizzy patient: symptomatic treatment of vertigo. *Postgrad Med*. 1983;73:317–324.
4. Baloh RW, Honrubia V, Jacobson K. Benign positional vertigo: clinical and oculographic features in 240 cases. *Neurology*. 1987;37:371–378.
5. Katsarkas A, Kirkham TH. Paroxysmal positional vertigo: a study of 255 cases. *J Otolaryngol*. 1978;7:320–330.
6. Schuknecht H, Ruby R. Cupulolithiasis. *Adv Otorhinolaryngol*. 1973; 20:434–443.
7. Baloh RW, Sakala SM, Honrubia V. Benign paroxysmal positional nystagmus. *Am J Otolaryngol*. 1979;1:1–5.
8. Harbert F. Benign paroxysmal positional nystagmus. *Arch Opththalmol*. 1970;84:298–302.
9. Alford B. Meniere's disease: criteria for diagnosis and evaluation of therapy for reporting: report of Subcommittee on Equilibrium and Measurement. *Trans Am Acad Ophthalmol Otolaryngol*. 1972;76:1462–1464.
10. Beal D. Effect of endolymphatic sac ablation in the rabbit and cat. *Acta Orolaryngol*. 1968;66:333–339.
11. Hallpike C, Cairns H. Observations on the pathology of Meniere's syndrome. *J Laryngol*. 1938;53:625–654.
12. Paparella MM. Pathology of Meniere's disease. *Ann Otol Rhinol Laryngol*. 1984;93(suppl 112):31–35.
13. Silverstein H. The effects of perfusing the perilymphatic space with artificial endolymph. *Ann Otol Rhinol Laryngol*. 1970;79:754–758.
14. Tumarkin I. Otolithic catastrophe: a new syndrome. *Brit Med J*. 1936;2:175–177.
15. Valvassori GE, Dobben GD. Multidirectional and computerized tomography of the vestibular aqueduct in Meniere's disease. *Ann Otol Rhinol Laryngol*. 1984;93:547–550.
16. Boles R, Rice DH, Hybels R, et al. Conservative management of Meniere's disease: Furstenberg regimen revisited. *Ann Otol Rhinol Laryngol*. 1975;84:513–517.
17. Jackson CG, et al. Medical management of Meniere's disease. *Ann Otol Rhinol Laryngol*. 1981;90:142–147.
18. Schuknecht HF. Endolymphatic hydrops: can it be controlled? *Ann Otol Rhinol Laryngol*. 1986;95:36–38.

19. Schuknecht HF, Kitamura RR, Nanfal PM. The pathology of idiopathic sensorineural hearing loss. *Arch Otorhinolaryngol.* 1986;243:1–9.

20. Zajtchuk J, Matz G, Lindsay J. Temporal bone pathology in herpes oticus. *Ann Otol Rhinol Laryngol.* 1972;81:331–336.

21. Grad A, Baloh RW. Vertigo of vascular origin: clinical and ENG features in 84 cases. *Arch Neurol.* 1989;46:281–285.

22. Waters EE, O'Connor PJ. Prevalence of migraine. *J Neurol Neurosurg Psychiatry.* 1975;38:613–616.

23. Kayan A, Hood JD. Neuro-otological manifestations of migraine. *Brain.* 1984;107: 1123–1142.

24. Harker LA, Rassek HC. Episodic vertigo in basilar migraine. *Otolaryngol Head Neck Surg.* 1987;96:239–250.

25. Prensky AL, Sommer D. Diagnosis and treatment of migraine in children. *Neurology.* 1979;29:506–510.

26. Diamond S, et al. Long-term study of propranolol in the treatment of migraine. *Headache.* 1982;22:268–271.

27. Ziegler DK, et al. Migraine prophylaxis: a comparison of propranolol and amitriptyline. *Arch Neurol.* 1987;44:486–489.

Motion Sickness

Kenneth L. Koch, MD

From the Argonauts of Greek myth to the astronauts of the space shuttle, a surprisingly high number of people have been affected by the syndrome of motion sickness. The ancient Greeks were probably first to associate the common symptoms of cold sweating, pallor, nausea, and vomiting with exposure to unfamiliar motion, whether real or illusory. Hippocrates wrote, "sailing on the sea proves that motion disorders the body," and the word "nausea" comes from the Greek *naus*, meaning ship. Some individuals, habituated to their symptoms, learn techniques for adapting to the debilitating effects of motion sickness. For others, depending on their susceptibility and the severity of movement to which they are exposed, the disorder can be a constant traveling companion.

As travel modes have changed dramatically over past decades, so have perceptions about the incidence of motion sickness and its etiology. Once thought to afflict only weak or neurotic individuals, motion sickness has affected approximately 90% of adults at some point in their lives. In one study based on a questionnaire, 57% of college students indicated that as children they had become nauseated when riding in cars and 32% remembered vomiting.[1] However, since many people adapt to motion in a car as they mature, their susceptibility to motion sickness in such vehicles is presumably outgrown by the time they reach adulthood. Certain travel settings are more conducive to motion sickness. For example, it is estimated that the incidence of motion sickness among passengers on ships crossing the Atlantic during moderate turbulence is 25% to 30% and that as many as 90% become sick under severe conditions.

Despite the prevalence of the syndrome, its long history, and a voluminous literature, previous misconceptions about the etiology of motion sickness led to considerable confusion about its pathophysiology. In the early literature, for example, vomiting is frequently referred to as a "vegetative" manifestation or as part of a series of autonomic responses to motion.[2] Yet the autonomic (visceral efferent) nerve supply to the gut is not needed for vomiting, which suggests that vomiting is not exclusively the result of activity in the autonomic nervous system. Nausea is commonly assumed to be the conscious awareness of unusual activity in the so-called vomiting centers, but in fact, this symptom is very poorly understood in pathophysiological terms.

Within the last 10 years, new concepts concerning the etiology of motion sickness have emerged. The most popular theory suggests that the pathophysiology is rooted in an organic, dynamic, and heterogenous process, earmarked by a neurosensory mismatch between the different systems responsible for spatial orientation. Recent laboratory investigations — including those using an optokinetic drum (Fig 1) in which healthy individuals are subjected to provocative stimuli that create an illusion of self-motion — have revealed more about the precise mechanisms involved in motion sickness.[3,4] Based on these data, it appears that:

(1) Motion sickness develops due to a sensory mismatch involving the visual, vestibular, and propioceptive systems.

(2) When sensory feedback from any of these systems is exaggerated and therefore not congruent with another, it triggers a series of neuroendocrine reactions and a complex chain of events beginning with activation of the sympathetic nervous system.

(3) Activation of the sympathetic nervous system correlates with the development of gastric dysrhythmias or tachyarrhythmias and increases in plasma epinephrine and norepinephrine.

(4) In response to appropriate physiological stimuli, vasopressin is secreted by the neurohypophysis, setting the stage for a hypothalamic-pituitary-gut interaction.

(5) Ultimately, the interactions among brain, gut, and increasing nausea reach a threshold that activates what is loosely referred to as the "vomiting center" located within the central nervous system. This vomiting center controls abdominal muscles, the respiratory system, and duodenal and gastric motility responsible for vomiting.

(6) When the "pattern generator" for vomiting is activated, reverse peristalsis and emesis occur; vomiting frequently relieves nausea, at least temporarily.

While this scheme represents an oversimplified, thumbnail sketch of the pathophysiology of motion-induced nausea and vomiting, recent literature has revealed more about the relative importance of these mechanisms and interactions and how they could influence the choice of therapy, either behavioral or pharmacologic.

Importance of the Vestibular System

The vestibular apparatus plays an indispensable role in the development of motion sickness and in some circumstances vestibular stimulation alone

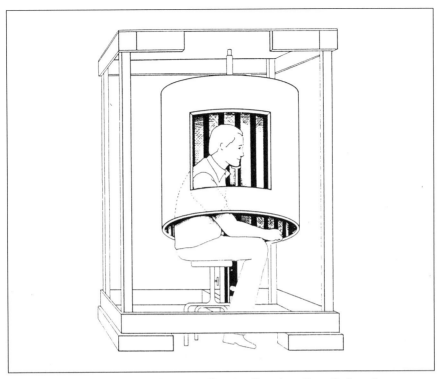

Fig 1. Circular vection drum used to create illusory self-motion. (From Koch et al. Neuroendocine and gastric myoelectrical responses to illusory self-motion in humans. *Am J Physiol.* 1990;258:E304-E310.)

may be the predisposing factor.[2] Are all people with normally functioning vestibular systems susceptible to motion sickness? Could it be that less susceptible people just require more of whatever it is that causes motion sickness in susceptible individuals? Early explanations for motion sickness included extreme movement of the viscera or overstimulation of the vestibular system. A more likely explanation is that it evolves from conflicting sensory inputs,[5] possibly from the vestibular system, the semicircular canals, and the otoliths. Most researchers point out that in a motion situation, the subject anticipates a particular set of sensory stimuli from the visual, vestibular, and, possibly, proprioceptive systems. Signals from these systems are normally closely related and congruent. When one or more of the sensory inputs do not conform to the expected pattern, a sensory mismatch occurs. These two examples illustrate how sensory mismatch may lead to motion sickness:

- A 2-year-old child sitting in the back seat of a car traveling on a winding road receives vestibular feedback that corresponds to the actual pattern of the car's movement. But because the child sees only the back of the front seat, the visual feedback indicates to him that there is little or no movement.

- An astronaut working in space has normal visual function, but head movements create new or unexpected sensory mismatches because the vestibular (otolith) system functions differently under conditions of zero gravity.

A striking demonstration of the importance of the vestibular apparatus comes from early literature in which several reports indicated that more than 70 deaf-mutes were immune to motion sickness during rough weather at sea. Other scattered reports in the literature confirm that immunity to motion sickness was evident in labyrinth-defective persons who were exposed to a slow-rotation room, storm conditions at sea, or aerobatics. Several studies in animal models confirm these observations, as investigators have shown that labyrinthectomy confers immunity to motion sickness. In some cases, vestibular stimulation per se can produce motion sickness. For example, while rotating at a constant angular velocity, periodic movement of the head about axes parallel to the plane of rotation is a strong stimulus of motion sickness in most blindfolded people. Although the importance of the vestibular apparatus is firmly established, it is still uncertain whether the otoliths or the semicircular canals of the inner ear, or both, are implicated in motion sickness. It appears, however, that under certain circumstances the semicircular canals are indispensable in the pathophysiology, while in other cases the otolith organs appear to be chiefly responsible.

Moving Visual Fields and Their Role in Motion Sickness

Despite the overriding importance assigned to the vestibular apparatus, neurosensory activity in two other systems also contributes to an individual's sense of orientation in three-dimensional space, in some cases providing conflicting sensory inputs that trigger motion sickness. Movement of the field of vision can cause all of the signs and symptoms of motion sickness because the illusion of motion that results conflicts with signals from the vestibular system. For example, flight simulators or large-screen movies often provoke motion sickness via visual stimuli.

A series of studies in the laboratory using a rotating optokinetic drum as a provocative stimulus demonstrates how moving visual fields create the classical sensory mismatches predisposing to motion sickness. Within a few seconds, all subjects experience vection—i.e., an illusion of self-motion—while neurosensory feedback from their vestibular and proprioceptive systems rightly indicates that they are sitting still. This sensory conflict provokes motion sickness in approximately 50% of unselected healthy human subjects.[5,6]

Laboratory experiments with the optokinetic drum have helped overcome one of the major obstacles to the prevention of motion sickness: the lack of quantifiable physiologic markers of the disorder. By quantifying changes in gastric myoelectric activity that accompany the onset of symptoms of motion sickness, we can determine how these markers correlate with, for example, alterations in the sympathetic nervous system and related neuroendocrine activity. Exploring the extent of these changes and their impact on brain-gut interactions may eventually allow us to tailor therapy more precisely and address the mechanisms of motion sickness at its earliest stages.

The Significance of Tachyarrhythmias

The optokinetic drum has enhanced our understanding of the mechanisms of motion sickness by providing a means to consistently and safely induce nausea. Vection is induced as the stationary subject gazes at vertical black-and-white stripes painted inside the rotating drum. When subjects are exposed to vection, symptoms of motion sickness—i.e., sweating, headache, dizziness, abdominal discomfort, and increasing intensity of nausea—develop in those who are susceptible.[3,6] Although most individuals who experience motion sickness describe symptoms of vague epigastric discomfort and nausea, the relationship between these symptoms and gastric motility has been largely neglected. Stern et al showed that vection produced symptoms of motion sickness in 14 of 21 subjects, and in each of the 14 the electrogastrograms (EGG), the frequency shifted from 3 cycles/min, which is normal, to 4–9 cycles/min, with frequencies which are abnormal, erratic patterns characteristic of tachyarrhythmias (Figs 2 and 3).[6] Although tachyarrhythmias are one of the most closely correlated variables with the symptoms of motion sickness, other physiological markers, including decreased mean successive differences of R-R intervals (RRI) and increased skin conductance levels, have also emerged as correlates.[7]

If compelling evidence points to an association between vection-induced tachygastria and motion sickness, what neurohormonal mechanisms are responsible for the gastric dysrhythmias? Although the answer is still unclear, some plausible and intriguing explanations have been posed. One theory stems from data indicating that sympathetic dominance accounts for gastric dysrhythmias after gastric surgery,[8] and that infusion of catecholamines, including dopamine, induces antral dysrhythmias

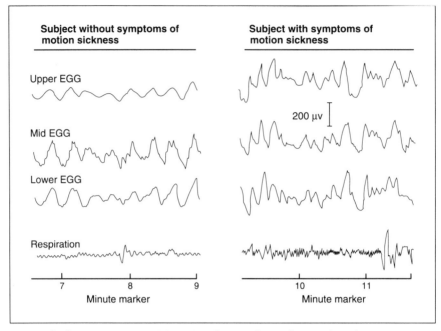

Fig 2. *Left,* electrogastrogram (EGG) tracings from a subject who experienced no symptoms of motion sickness and remained in normal 3 cycles/min rhythm. *Right,* EGG in a subject who became sick and requested that the drum be stopped at minute 11. Note the development of tachyarrhythmia of 5–7 cycles/min prior to the symptoms of motion sickness. (From Stern RM, et al. Tachygastria and motion sickness. *Aviat Space Environ Med.* 1985;56:1074–1077.)

in dogs.[9] It suggests that the "stress" of vection and the resulting visual-vestibular-propioceptive mismatch causes a release of catecholamines, which temporarily suppresses or overwhelms gastric vagal input and precipitates gastric tachyarrhythmias. The onset of tachyarrhythmias typically precedes the first reports of nausea by 2 to 3 minutes. Thus, the shift from normal 3 cycles/min gastric rhythms to tachyarrhythmias is a physiological antecedent of nausea and motion sickness.[10]

Utilizing running spectral analysis, a relatively new method of quantifying gastric dysrhythmias, Stern et al showed several distinct EGG frequency peaks (Fig 4) in the tachygastria range during motion sickness symptoms, indicating instability of the slow-wave pacemaker and suggesting the possibility of multiple and/or wandering pacemaker foci.[11]

To what extent, then, is vection a stressful stimulus? If subjects do not develop motion sickness during vection, can we conclude that vection elicits minimal activity of sympathetic or humoral pathways which might disturb slow-wave rhythm? Symptom-free subjects do in fact maintain gastric rhythms of 3 cycles/min and do not develop increases in catecholamines or cortisol levels.[3] Nor do they develop changes in parasympathetic vagal ac-

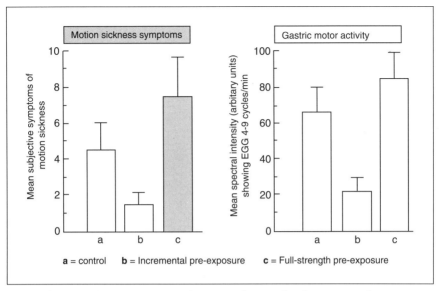

Fig 3. *Left*, mean subjective symptoms of motion sickness and *Right*, intensity of gastric tachyarrhythmia. (EGG 4–9 cycles/min) during rotation at 10 revolutions/min. a, control subjects; b, subjects who had brief periods of exposure to gradually increasing speed of drum rotation, from 2.5 to 5 revolutions/min prior to the test period; c, subjects who beforehand, had brief periods of exposure at the same high speed as in the test period (10 revolutions/min). Note the large attenuation of reported symptoms and of tachyarrhythmia in the incremental pre-exposure group. (Redrawn from Hu S, Grant WF, Stern RM, Koch KL. Motion sickness severity and physiological correlates during repeated exposures to a rotating optokinetic drum. *Aviat Space Environ Med.* 1991;62:308–314.)

tivity. On the other hand, once the stress of vection is removed in symptomatic subjects, the normal 3 cycles/min EGG pattern returns, suggesting the restoration of baseline conditions or sympathetic-parasympathetic balance.

The Significance of Heart Rate and Skin Conductance

More extensive use of the optokinetic drum has also enabled investigators to explore whether other physiological markers—such as heart rate and skin conductance level—change in response to motion sickness. There has been wide disagreement on this issue as investigators have measured heart rate variability by calculating the coefficient of variance (CV) of RRI, i.e., the variability in successive interbeat intervals. By exploring these relationships, more can be learned about the role of sympathetic nervous system activity in the appearance of gastric tachyarrhythmia and symptoms of motion sickness. The most recent study[7] showed, for example, that although mean heart rate increased during the drum rotation period, the differences among groups based on severity of symptoms were not

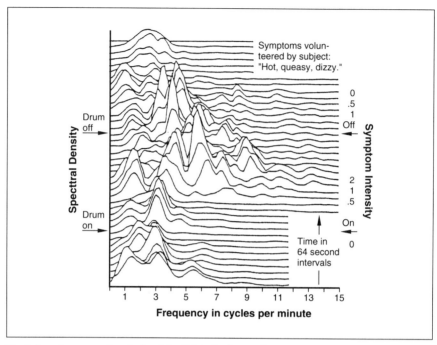

Fig 4. Running spectral analysis of the EGG of subject who reported sweating, dizziness, and a queasy stomach during rotation. Whereas 3- and 1- cycle/min activity dominates the spectral analysis before drum rotation, 6 minutes after the onset of rotation, spectral density showed a peak of 6 cycles/min, with additional activity in the tachygastria range (5–9 cycles/min). At approximately this point the subject reported his first symptoms of motion sickness. (From Stern RM et al. Spectral analysis of tachygastria recorded during motion sickness. *Gastroenterology.* 1987;93:92–97.)

statistically significant. Consequently, increases in heart rate cannot be used as a sensitive marker of motion-sickness susceptibility.

In contrast, a decrease in variability of heart rate—represented by reductions in the mean successive differences of RRI—was significantly correlated with a *decrease* in parasympathetic activity or vagal tone and the development of motion sickness. These successive differences, reflecting the beat-to-beat variation in RRI were important markers of changes in parasympathetic tone. The high correlation between the reduction of mean successive differences of RRI and the increase in motion sickness severity showed that the development of motion sickness was accompanied by *vagal withdrawal.* These findings, when coupled with results suggesting that skin conductance increased in relation to the severity of motion sickness symptoms, strengthen the theory that increased sympathetic nervous system activity is an important factor in the onset of motion sickness. It appears that in subjects who develop motion sickness as sympathetic activity increases and parasympathetic activity decreases, autonomic nervous system "balance" is perturbed soon after initial exposure to vection. These changes are thought to underlie the shift to gastric tachyarrhythmias preceding the onset of nausea.

The disclosure that tachyarrhythmias are physiological markers correlating with symptoms of motion sickness is important because we no longer need to depend solely on a patient's subjective interpretation of epigastric distress or nausea. It should be noted, however, that tachyarrhythmias do not indicate faster muscular activity in the stomach. Rather, they refer to erratic, rapid, electrical discharges from the neuromuscular apparatus of the stomach antrum independent of gastric contractions. Patients who suffer from nausea because of diabetic gastroparesis,[12] pregnancy,[13] or unexplained nausea conditions all show EGG recordings reflecting these gastric dysrhythmias. This intriguing finding could bring us closer to identifying the basic mechanisms underlying nausea, thus enabling development of more accurately directed therapeutic approaches to correct the dysrhythmias and accompanying symptoms.

Neuroendocrine Responses During Motion Sickness

Although postvagotomy dysrhythmias are attributed to "sympathetic dominance," the underlying mechanisms of human gastric dysrhythmias are unknown. Glucagon, a gut hormone, precipitated gastric dysrhythmias and nausea when administered to healthy volunteers and dogs. As mentioned above, infusions of epinephrine and Met-enkephalin also induced gastric dysrhythmias in dogs, indicating that adrenergic and opioid pathways may mediate the dysrhythmias.[9]

Recent research has brought us a step closer to understanding sympathetic nervous system involvement in motion sickness by identifying gastric and neuroendocrine correlates of the disorder. A recent study by Koch et al measured catecholamines, cortisol, and beta-endorphin fluxes in healthy subjects who either did or did not develop motion sickness elicited by vection.[3] As expected, their study found that norepinephrine was increased transiently 1 minute after drum rotation stopped, at which time nausea and gastric dysrhythmias were present. In subjects with motion sickness, epinephrine levels after vection also were significantly elevated compared with baseline values. In contrast, norepinephrine and epinephrine levels did not change in asymptomatic subjects, some of whom actually found the motion stimuli exhilarating. Their unchanged epinephrine, norepinephrine, and cortisol levels during the drum ride indicate that they were not stressed by illusory motion. Could these subjects be thrill-seekers who love speed, are willing to stand in long lines for roller coaster rides, and might someday volunteer as civilians in space?

The neuroendocrine responses to vection among the symptomatic group indicated that extra-adrenal sympathetic neurons and the sympathoadrenomedullary system were significantly stimulated[3]—a revealing finding consistent with previous reports, including those that studied motion sickness induced by a rotary chair.[14] Such results reinforced the impression that activation of the sympathetic nervous system may help to mediate gastric dysrhythmias during motion sickness.

Searching for corroborating evidence, we suspected that plasma dopamine also would increase in subjects who had vection-induced motion sickness and tachyarrhythmias. Previous studies had laid the groundwork for this assumption by showing that dopamine infusions decrease intragastric pressure, elicit retching and vomiting, and cause gastric dysrhythmias in dogs. Several reports demonstrated, too, that gastric tone and peristalsis are decreased and liquid emptying delayed in subjects who experience motion sickness induced by swings and rotating-chair stimuli. However, the absence of a consistent pattern of dopamine levels in nauseated subjects[3] has led researchers to believe that endogenous dopamine levels are not crucial in the development of nausea and gastric tachyarrhythmias elicited by vection. These dopamine data may explain why dopamine receptor antagonists do not reduce motion sickness induced by space travel or rotating chairs.

Cortisol was increased in response to a variety of stressful stimuli, including the stress of severe exercise and surgical operations. Increases in cortisol are stimulated principally by pituitary adrenocorticotropic hormone (ACTH), which, in turn, is stimulated by corticotropin-releasing factor (CRF), a hypothalamic neuropeptide that integrates the body's hypothalamic-pituitary-adrenal and sympathetic and parasympathetic nervous system responses to stress. Baseline cortisol levels rose in those subjects who went on to develop motion sickness during vection, but because baseline catecholamine levels were similar in symptomatic and asymptomatic subjects, this increase could not be attributed to catecholamine effects on ACTH release. We concluded that the increased baseline cortisol levels in the motion sickness group measured 15 minutes *before* drum rotation began were due to enhanced ACTH (and CRF) release and were related to the anticipation and anxiety produced by the imminent motion stimulus.

Anticipatory cortisol responses may be an important factor in determining why susceptible subjects developed vection-induced gastric dysrhythmias and nausea. Fasting gastric motility patterns are inhibited by intracerebroventricular injections of cortisol, ACTH, and CRF in dogs. Animal models suggest, too, that CRF effects on gastric motility are independent of pituitary and adrenal activity and appear to involve the noradrenergic nervous system and opioid pathways.[15] Corticotropin-releasing factor also stimulates sympathetic nervous system activity and the release of norepinephrine and epinephrine.[16] Thus, CRF-stimulated pituitary-adrenal axis activity during the baseline period may have lowered the threshold for vection-induced gastric tachyarrhythmias and motion sickness, raising the question of whether anticipatory nausea related to chemotherapy or other situations might also be mediated by these pathways.

Healthy subjects who developed symptoms of motion sickness demonstrated other anticipatory neurohormonal responses. Baseline beta-endorphin levels 15 minutes before drum rotation were significantly greater in subjects who subsequently became motion sick. Anticipation of queasiness inside the rotating drum was already triggering a cascade of central nervous system responses in these subjects. Because ACTH and beta-endorphin are derived from a common precursor, proopiolipomelanocortin, these results further suggest involvement of the anterior pituitary in the anticipatory responses to vection. Moreover, CRF is again implicated indirectly in these responses because this peptide releases beta-endorphin and ACTH from the pituitary.

Interestingly, the sustained increases in epinephrine and cortisol observed later in the *recovery period* in subjects with motion sickness are similar to the delayed catecholamine and cortisol responses induced by the stress of strenuous exercise in untrained healthy individuals. The sustained epinephrine levels and the increasing cortisol and beta-endorphin levels in nauseated subjects during the recovery period probably reflect the neuroendocrine responses to the stress of the symptoms of motion sickness rather than to vection per se. In contrast, asymptomatic subjects did not show significant catecholamine, cortisol, or beta-endorphin responses during vection. Thus, the symptomatic subjects exhibited *anticipatory* hypercortisolism *and* a sustained increase in cortisol after motion sickness, indicating the stress response to the motion sickness itself.

To summarize, three interrelated stages of neuroendocrine activity were observed in patients with motion sickness:

(1) Anticipatory activation of the pituitary-adrenocortical axis (as shown by the cortisol and beta-endorphin response during baseline);

(2) Increased activity of the nonadrenal sympathetic nervous system and sympathoadrenomedullary pathways during nausea and gastric tachyarrhythmias (as reflected in the increased norepinephrine and epinephrine responses at 1 minute); and

(3) Sympathoadrenomedullary and pituitary-adrenocortical axis activity during recovery (demonstrated by epinephrine, cortisol, and beta-endorphin responses later in the recovery period after vection).

These profound changes in sympathetic nervous system and hypothalamic-pituitary-adrenal axis activity ultimately affect the key peripheral target—the stomach—as reflected in the shift to gastric tachyarrhythmias beginning early after vection in association with nausea. This brain-gut interaction becomes stronger, perhaps modulated and reinforced by the changes in stomach rhythm until motion sickness and nausea become more severe, culminating in vomiting.

Vasopressin Response and Its Role in Motion Sickness

Motion sickness is fatiguing, even debilitating—a situation clearly different from the classic "fight-or-flight" response associated with activation of the sympathoadrenal systems. Therefore, other pathways and mechanisms must be operative in motion sickness and nausea. It has been speculated that vasopressin—a nonapeptide synthesized in magnocellular and parvicellular neurons in the paraventricular and supraoptic nuclei of the hypothalamus—is released by nausea.

Since vasopressin release is stimulated by ingestion of water, apomorphine,[17] and chemotherapy,[18] we postulated that vasopressin secretion would also be elevated when healthy subjects were exposed to the illusion of self-motion. If nausea reported during motion sickness were associated with the release of vasopressin, another piece of the puzzle would be at hand, since vasopressin secretion originates in hypothalamic nuclei where sympathetic and parasympathetic controls are located.

We studied 12 healthy volunteers, none of whom had a history of gastrointestinal, vestibular, or central nervous system disorders, by subjecting them to the optokinetic drum. Blood was sampled to determine vasopressin levels. A significant increase in vasopressin levels was observed in subjects who developed nausea and gastric dysrhythmias during vection (mean, 35.4 pmol/L) compared with asymptomatic subjects (mean, 2.7 pmol/L) (Fig 5).

Thus, the purely optokinetic stimuli that produces illusory self-motion will release vasopressin in susceptible individuals with nausea. Although it is not known whether nausea stimulates vasopressin production or whether release of vasopressin stimulates nausea, evidence is mounting for an association between the two.

Nausea and Motion Sickness:
A Brain-Gut/Gut-Brain Interaction

When susceptible individuals experience or anticipate a neurosensory mismatch involving motion, or vection, the consequent stress evokes increased

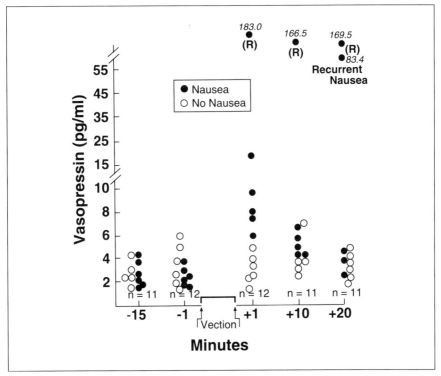

Fig 5. Vasopressin responses to vection in subjects with and without nausea and gastric dysrhythmias. Baseline values were similar in the two groups of subjects. Mean vasopressin values at 1 minute were increased significantly ($P < 0.05$) in subjects with nausea and were significantly greater ($P < 0.05$) than those in subjects with no nausea. One subject retched (R) immediately before the drum was stopped, and one subject had a recurrence of nausea during the recovery period. (From Koch KL, Summy-Long J, Bingaman S, Sperry N, Stern RM. Vasopressin and oxytocin responses to illusory self-motion and nausea in man. *J Clin Endocrinol Metab.* 1990;71:1269–1275.)

sympathetic nervous system activity, which in turn leads to a shift from normal 3 cycles/minute gastric electrical activity to tachyarrhythmias—a brain-gut interaction. Disruption of the stomach is monitored by the central nervous system via vagal or splanchnic afferent nerves. The ongoing gastric dysrhythmias may in part affect hypothalamic vasopressinergic nuclei which release vasopressin from the posterior pituitary—a gut-brain interaction. Thus, the presence of gastric dysrhythmias, as well as increased sympathetic and vasopressinergic activity, result in the progression of motion sickness symptoms from sweating to severe nausea.

At the stage of severe nausea, the pattern generator for vomiting is activated in the "vomiting center"—a term coined 25 years ago to describe a stereotyped program within the brain stem that controls activity of the abdominal muscles, duodenum, stomach, and esophagus required for vomiting. Once the vomiting reflex is activated, reverse peristalsis beginning in the duodenum is initiated and continues through the stomach, forcing gastric contents through the relaxed esophagus and mouth.

Treatment

Behavioral Adaptation and Techniques

As mentioned above in regard to children and car sickness, re-exposures to the motion stimulus will often lead to adaptation and lessening of symptoms. The same is true for re-exposures to air or sea travel. Similarly, when subjects were exposed to the rotating optokinetic drum for three sessions with relatively brief intervals (less than 48 hours) between them, symptoms and physiologic changes were decreased.[19] However, subjects did *not* adapt if the intervals were longer. These findings suggest that adaptation may be helped by gradually increasing the frequency of exposure to the motion stimulus. Whether the adaptation to vection confers resistance to other motion stimuli is not known.

Older reports indicate that in some vehicles the benefits of lying in the supine position are probably at least equal to those of drugs commonly used for motion sickness. The incidence of sickness in this position has been reported to be as low as one fifth of the incidence in the sitting position. Intermittent recumbency, which can be combined with drug therapy, is an effective measure in some cases. On ships, trains, or vehicles that simulate swinging motion, susceptible individuals may benefit from lying flat on the back with only a thin pillow.

Considerable evidence indicates that minimizing body movement, particularly head movement, is beneficial. For example, there were few reports of motion sickness from the first space flights when the capsules were so small that the astronauts could hardly move. Space sickness emerged when large vehicles like the shuttle required astronauts to move among various work areas.

In rotating rooms, restricting head movement to eliminate sensory mismatch is completely effective in preventing sickness. In vehicles with a high-backed seat, sufficient restriction of head movement to overcome motion sickness is often gained by simply holding the head against the back of the seat. Even when this is not possible, restriction of head movement can be voluntary. Patients should be warned to move the head slowly and only when necessary.

Another school of thought focuses on visual orientation as an important factor in preventing symptoms. Individuals are urged to look at the movement that is simultaneously stimulating their vestibular organs during travel. For example, looking out the window of a car at a fixed point in the distance while being driven on a winding road may be helpful, as the visual system stabilizes the movement relative to the vestibular stimulation. Likewise, victims of seasickness can experience relief by walking on deck and viewing the distant horizon. When below deck and during turbulence, however, it is advisable to keep the eyes closed, in which case it is especially important to restrain movements of the head.

Eating

Despite the conventional wisdom that travelers susceptible to air sickness should refrain from eating before their trip, scientific evidence suggests that food may in fact suppress the symptoms of motion sickness.[20] In a study on the effects of eating on vection-induced motion sickness all subjects reported to the laboratory the morning after an overnight fast. One group was given fruit juice, cold cereal with milk, and a doughnut, while the other group read a newspaper. Compared with the fasted group, the fed group showed enhanced respiratory sinus arrhythmia (i.e., increased parasympathetic tone), increased gastric activity at the normal rate of 3 cycles/minute, and less gastric dysrhythmia. This group also reported fewer symptoms of motion sickness during vection. Consequently, it appears that meal-induced increases in parasympathetic activity and normal gastric myoelectric activity can alleviate motion sickness partly by suppressing gastric dysrhythmias. A light meal consisting primarily of carbohydrates may be eaten before exposure to motion stimuli to prevent gastric dysrhythmias and nausea.

Drug Treatment

Gastric and neuroendocrine changes during motion sickness have provided investigators with new insights in developing strategies to treat and prevent nausea and other symptoms of motion sickness. For example, the fact that similar gastric dysrhythmias are found in patients with chronic nausea and in healthy subjects with motion sickness suggests that treatment may be aimed at converting gastric dysrhythmia to the normal 3 cycles/minute. A study in diabetics with nausea showed that this pharmacologic "gastroversion" is a possibility.[12] Neuroendocrine changes during motion sickness suggest that adrenergic blockade may be useful; and vasopressin antagonists may also ameliorate nausea and motion sickness. Thus far, though, no studies have been undertaken to test these strategies. Ongoing investigations are focusing on circuits that control release of vasopressin. Among the questions being addressed: Are serotonin or opioid pathways involved in controlling relevant motion sickness circuits?

At present, a relatively small number of agents currently comprise the drugs of choice. Pharmacologic therapy is anchored by scopolamine, which has been used for treating motion sickness since the late 1940s. By avoiding the relatively high concentration of scopolamine in the blood that occurs after oral or intramuscular administration, transdermal administration of scopolamine (Fig 6) has helped reduce the incidence of side effects, including extreme fatigue, dryness of the mouth, and blurred vision.[21] The transdermal delivery system requires only one fourth of the oral dose to achieve the same reduction in symptoms.[21] Studies have documented protection ranging from 60% to 80%, depending on the severity of motion. Bioavailability studies indicate that absorption from the posterior auricular area is greater than from any other body area tested except for the scrotum. Bioavailability is also maintained for a relatively long period because blood levels approximately 12 hours after application of the transdermal system reflected essentially constant scopolamine levels until removal of the patch 60 hours later.

Timing is the key factor in the efficacy of the transdermal therapeutic system scopolamine (TTSS). Application of a scopolamine patch in the posterior auricular area less than 4 hours prior to sea travel, for example, results in a significantly higher incidence of motion sickness than if the patch is applied 8 or more hours prior to the voyage. Although the precise mechanisms of scopolamine's effectiveness are not known, it is believed that the drug's anticholinergic activity antagonizes the parasympathetic system, thereby preventing vomiting. Recent studies have demonstrated that low doses of scopolamine increase parasympathetic tone and reduce nausea and tachygastria when administered to subjects exposed to vection (Uijtdehaage SHJ, Stern RM, Koch KL, unpublished data).

In addition to scopolamine, dimenhydrinate is the other mainstay of motion sickness therapy,[22] although many more drugs have been tested empirically. Dimenhydrinate is believed to be effective in preventing nausea and vomiting because it antagonizes histamine receptors. However, in a recent comparison with transdermal scopolamine, dimenhydrinate was not as effective in reducing the incidence of motion sickness. Overall, transdermal scopolamine protected 62% of subjects from motion sickness at sea compared with 49% of those treated with dimenhydrinate.[23]

In rotating chair–induced motion sickness, a number of amphetamines have been shown to reduce motion sickness,[24] but these have not been tried in other forms of the syndrome. Dilantin is an untested but potentially useful medication.[25] The protective effect of scopolamine in most studies ranges from 60% to 80%, leaving room for the next generation of drugs to improve those rates and address the needs of the 20% to 40% of patients

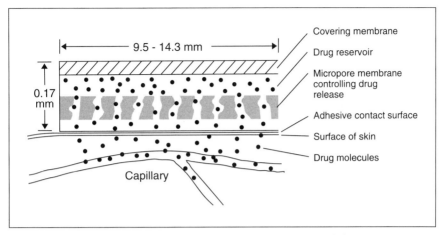

Fig 6. Transdermal therapeutic system. (From Noy S, et al. Transdermal therapeutic system scopolamine (TTSS), dimenhydrate, and placebo: a comparative study at sea. *Aviat Space Environ Med.* 1984;55:1051–1054.)

whose disorder may be refractory to conventional treatment. Alternatively, nonpharmacologic approaches such as diet and adaptation programs[26] may prove useful with or without concommitant drug therapy. It is hoped that insight gained from the study of motion sickness will eventually lead to a fuller understanding of the physiological mechanisms of nausea, and in the process yield a more rational approach to its treatment in a variety of clinical settings.

References

1. Lawther A, Griffin MJ. The motion of a ship at sea and the consequent motion sickness amongst passengers. *Ergonomics.* 1986;29:535–552.
2. Money KE. Motion sickness. *Physiol Rev.* 1970;50(1):1–30.
3. Koch KL, Stern RM, Vasey MW, Seaton JF, Demers LM, Harrison TS. Neuroendocrine and gastric myoelectrical responses to illusory self-motion in humans. *Am J Physiol.* 1990;258:E304-E310.
4. Koch KL, Summy-Long J, Bingaman S, Sperry N, Stern RM. Vasopressin and oxytocin responses to illusory self-motion and nausea in man. *J Clin Endocrinol Metab.* 1990;71:1269–1275.
5. Reason JT. Motion sickness adaptation: a neural mismatch model. *J Royal Soc Med.* 1978;71:819–829.
6. Stern RM, Koch KL, Leibowitz HW, Lindblad MS, Shupert CL, Stewart WR. Tachygastria and motion sickness. *Aviat Space Environ Med.* 1985;56:1074–1077.
7. Hu S, Grant WF, Stern RM, Koch KL. Motion sickness severity and physiological correlates during repeated exposures to a rotating optokinetic drum. *Aviat Space Environ Med.* 1991;62:308–314.
8. Stoddard CJ, Smallwood RH, Duthie HL. Electrical arrhythmias in the human stomach. *Gut.* 1981;92:993–999.

9. Kim CH, Zionsmeister AR, Malagelada J-R. Mechanisms of canine gastric dysrhythmias. *Gastroenterology.* 1987;92:993–999.

10. Koch KL, Stern RM, Summy-Long J, Bingaman S, Sperry N. Gastric dysrhythmias precede activation of vasopressinergic pathways during vection-induced nausea in man. *J Gastrointest Motil.* 1989;1:53.

11. Stern RM, Koch KL, Stewart WR, Lindblad IM. Spectral analysis of tachygastria recorded during motion sickness. *Gastroenterology.* 1987;93:92–97.

12. Koch KL, Stern RM, Stewart WR, Vasey MW, Sullivan ML. Gastric emptying and gastric myoelectrical activity in patients with symptomatic diabetic gastroparesis: effect of long-term domperidone treatment. *Am J Gastroenterol.* 1989;84:1069–1075.

13. Koch KL, Stern RM, Vasey M, Botti JJ, Creasy GW, Dwyer A. Gastric dysrhythmias and nausea of pregnancy. *Dig Dis Sci.* 1990;35:961–968.

14. Cowings PS, Suter S, Toscano WB, Kamiya J, Naifeh K. General autonomic components of motion sickness. *Psychophysiology.* 1986;23:542–551.

15. Lenz HJ, Burlage M, Raedler A, Greten H. Central nervous system effects of corticotropin-releasing factor: actions on the sympathetic nervous system and metabolism. *Endocrinology.* 1982;111:928–931.

16. Brown MR, Fisher LA, Spiess J, Rivier C, Rivier J, Vale W. Corticotropin-releasing factor: actions on the sympathetic nervous system and metabolism. *Endocrinology.* 1982;111:928–931.

17. Feldman M, Samson WK, O'Dorisio TM. Apomorphine-induced nausea in humans: release of vasopressin and pancreatic polypeptide. *Gastroenterology.* 1988;95:721–726.

18. Fisher RD, Rentschler RE, Nelson JC, Godfrey TE, Wilbur DW. Elevation of plasma antidiuretic hormone (ADH) associated with chemotherapy-induced emesis in man. *Cancer Treat Rep.* 1982;66:25–29.

19. Stern RM, Hu S, Vasey MW, Koch KL. Adaptation to vection-induced symptoms of motion sickness. *Aviat Space Environ Med.* 1989;60:566–572.

20. Uijtdehaage SHJ, Stern RM, Koch KL. Effects of eating on vection-induced motion sickness, cardiac vagal tone and gastric myoelectrical activity. *Psychophysiology.* 1992;29:193–201.

21. Levy GD, Rapaport MH. Transderm scopolamine efficacy related to time of application prior to the onset of motion. *Aviat Space Environ Med.* 1985;56:591–593.

22. Wood CD, Graybiel A. Evaluation of sixteen anti-motion sickness drugs under controlled laboratory conditions. *Aerospace Med.* 1968;39:1341–1344.

23. Noy S, Shapira S, Zilbiger A, Ribak J. Transdermal therapeutic system scopolamine (TTSS), dimenhydrate, and placebo: a comparative study at sea. *Aviat Space Environ Med.* 1984;55:1051–1054.

24. Kohl RL, Calkins DS, Mandell AJ. Arousal and stability: the effects of five new sympathomimetic drugs suggest a new principle for the prevention of space motion sickness. *Aviat Space Environ Med.* 1986;57:137–143.

25. Muth ER, Uijtdehaage SHJ, Stern RM, Koch KL. Effects of phenytoin on vection-induced motion sickness and gastric myoelectric activity. *Gastroenterology.* 1992;102:A937.

26. Hu S, Stern RM, Koch KL. Electrical acustimulation relieves vection-induced motion sickness. *Gastroenterology.* 1992;102:1854–1858.

Gastrointestinal Motility Disorders

Sidney F. Phillips, MD

The gut is often suspected of being the cause of unexplained nausea and vomiting. The diagnostic challenge lies in pinpointing which of many potential gastrointestinal mechanisms is the specific cause of these symptoms.[1] The extensive list of possible mechanisms responsible for nausea and vomiting includes mechanical obstruction at any level of the gut, inflammation and other structural diseases (especially of the proximal gut), dysmotility syndromes, and psychogenic disorders (Table 1).

Mechanical obstruction at the level of the stomach or intestines usually is accompanied by nausea and vomiting. If the obstruction is incomplete, other classic symptoms (pain) and signs (distention) may not develop completely, and the diagnosis may be missed. Inflammation and ulceration, especially in the proximal tract, also may present as recurrent vomiting without pain. Peritonitis from any cause can also result in vomiting by reflex mechanisms. Further complicating the differential diagnosis of nausea and vomiting is a wide range of neuromuscular disorders, including diseases of the central nervous system or those involving the nerves or smooth muscle of the gut. Diabetes mellitus may cause gastroparesis, which often presents as recurrent vomiting. Also high on the list of other illnesses to exclude—considering their growing incidence—are psychogenic disorders.

Pathologic vomiting, even when repetitive, may be a conscious and voluntary act, as it is in patients with bulimia, who vomit in part to control their weight.[1] In rumination, a related phenomenon, the patient increases intra-abdominal pressure, regurgitates food into the mouth, and swallows it again.[2,3] At a more subconscious level, vomiting may occur in otherwise healthy persons as part of a strong emotional reaction. Vomiting in neurotic patients may be an expression of an underlying psychopathologic condition, such as a conversion reaction.[3,4] Because of the broad spectrum of psychogenic disorders in which unexplained nausea and vomiting may be a presenting feature, the clinician needs to explore this possibility.

Table 1. Classification of Illnesses That Cause Nausea and Vomiting

Mechanical obstruction in the gastrointestinal tract: intraluminal, mural, extrinsic

Structural nonobstructive disease of the gut

    Mucosal lesion in stomach or duodenum, such as ulcer, inflammation, atrophy

    Pancreatic or small intestinal diseases

    Diseases of components of the gut wall

        Collagen, such as scleroderma

        Smooth muscle, such as hollow visceral myopathy, amyloidosis

        Nerve, such as chronic idiopathic intestinal pseudo-obstruction

Metabolic and endocrine diseases, such as uremia, diabetic ketoacidosis, adrenal insufficiency, hyperparathyroidism, pregnancy

Alterations in neural control of gut motility

    Diseases that affect one of the levels of neural control

    Diseases that affect neural reflexes, such as drug intoxication, labyrinthine diseases, migraine, cardiac vomiting

    Drugs affecting extrinsic autonomic supply, such as anticholinergic or adrenergic agents

Psychiatric disease: rumination, bulimia, anorexia nervosa

From Malagelada J-R, Camilleri MV. Unexplained vomiting: a diagnostic challenge. *Ann Intern Med.* 1984;101:211–218.

Gastrointestinal Mechanisms for Chronic Nausea and Vomiting

Mechanical Obstruction

The most important task for the physician caring for a patient with nausea and vomiting is to verify or exclude a mechanical obstruction of the gut. Mechanical obstruction will usually necessitate surgery, rather than treatment by medications. The key evaluations are plain abdominal x-rays, endoscopy, and barium x-ray studies of the gastrointestinal tract.

Inflammation and Other Structural Disorders

Inflammation or ulceration of the esophagus, stomach, or duodenum is a frequent cause of nausea and sometimes leads to vomiting. These conditions are usually accompanied by pain, often with characteristics that suggest the diagnosis. The most common cause of inflammation and ulceration in these regions is acid peptic disease. Acid regurgitation, with gastroesophageal reflux, leads to esophageal inflammation and ulceration. The other common manifestations of acid peptic disease are ulcerations in the stomach or in the first part of the duodenum. The clinician should be particularly alert to peptic ulceration in the pyloric canal, a condition often difficult to diagnose by radiology or endoscopy. Ulceration in the pylorus produces less pain than ulceration in other regions; thus, the patient may present with nausea and vomiting but with little of the pain usually associated with peptic ulcer disease.

Etiologic factors other than acid peptic disease need to be considered as potential causes of inflammation and ulceration in the upper gut. Esophagitis can be caused by infections with agents such as herpes simplex virus or Candida. Infection of the stomach with *Helicobacter pylori* is now recognized as a common cause of gastritis, and the dyspepsia and nausea may be severe enough to induce vomiting.

Gastric inflammation and ulceration are often associated with the use of medications, and side effects of medications must always be kept in mind as a possible cause of nausea and vomiting. When surgery has been performed on the stomach, often because of peptic ulcer disease, intestinal fluids (bile and pancreatic juice) may reflux into the stomach, where they can cause inflammation and ulceration. Abdominal discomfort, nausea, esophageal reflux, and vomiting may result.

The most dramatic example of inflammation and ulceration of the upper digestive tract is seen in Zollinger-Ellison syndrome. Gross hypersecretion of acid can lead to inflammation that may extend from the esophagus to the distal duodenum. Although pain is often present, nausea and vomiting may be the primary manifestations. Inflammation and ulceration in these regions can cause partial obstruction of the bowel because of edematous swelling; pyloric stenosis is the most common example. In these instances, persistent vomiting will be the usual manifestation.

Esophageal Motility Disorders

Gastroesophageal reflux. Unexplained nausea and vomiting may be due to altered motility of the upper gut. Thus, patients with upper gastrointestinal symptoms may need to be managed by measures other than those aimed at controlling secretion.

Although treatment of gastroesophageal reflux disease tends to focus on efforts to suppress acid, there is no evidence that patients with this disorder are hypersecreters.[5] Patients with chronic reflux tend to have comparatively weak esophageal contractions and reduced pressures at the lower sphincter, suggesting that a motility component may contribute to the disease. It is unclear, however, whether a motility abnormality is the cause or the result of reflux. If reflux disease is primarily a problem of abnormal motility, advisable treatment may be with drugs that enhance motility, increase esophageal contraction and sphincteric pressures, or correct delayed gastric emptying.

Achalasia. Achalasia is characterized variably by aperistalsis of the esophagus, elevated resting lower esophageal sphincter pressure, failure of the lower esophageal sphincter to relax completely, and esophageal dilatation.[6] The manometric diagnosis is rather precise. Clinically, the predominant symptom of achalasia is dysphagia; patients experience difficulty in swallowing both solids and liquids. Weight loss, vomiting (usually without nausea), and regurgitation of esophageal contents are common. Pulmonary disease frequently results from repeated, insidious aspiration of regurgitated esophageal contents. Treatment is surgical (Heller's myotomy) or endoscopic (forceful dilatation).

Other Disorders

Chagas' disease is seen mainly in South American countries. Neural degeneration results from a toxin elaborated by *Trypanosoma cruzi* and causes esophageal aperistalsis.

In other esophageal disorders, nonspecific abnormal contractile patterns may be seen. Diffuse esophageal spasm is characterized by powerful simultaneous contractions and intermittent normal peristalsis. So-called "nutcracker esophagus" is a condition featuring greatly increased amplitudes of normal peristalsis. Hypertensive lower esophageal sphincter (LES) is a disorder characterized by elevated LES pressure but normal LES relaxation. Treatment of this heterogeneous group of conditions is medical.

Gastroparesis and Intestinal Pseudo-Obstruction

Gastroparesis. Although it is probably quite common, postviral gastroparesis has been clearly described in only a few anecdotal case reports. A recent study at the Mayo Clinic[7] described the clinical features and long-term outcome of seven patients who had gastroparesis after a presumed viral illness. All seven developed persistent nausea, vomiting, and epigastric pain a mean of 4.5 days after the spontaneous resolution of the viral illness. In all patients, delayed emptying of gastric contents was substantiated. The authors advise that postviral gastroparesis should be suspected in young persons with symptoms of gastric stasis, such as nausea, vomiting, and epigastric discomfort, after an influenza-like illness.

An autonomic neuropathy is sometimes noted in patients with postviral gastroparesis.[7] It can be detected by changes in blood pressure in the supine and upright positions or by variations in the RR interval on electrocardiograms in response to Valsalva deep-breathing maneuvers.

Intestinal pseudo-obstruction. Intestinal pseudo-obstruction consists of a group of syndromes resulting from impairment of gut motility.[8] It is classified as either acute or chronic.

Acute pseudo-obstruction is most often manifested as an isolated colonic disturbance. It tends to be associated with significant extraintestinal conditions.[8] Most frequently colonic pseudo-obstruction (Ogilvie's syndrome) occurs in hospitalized patients, as a complication of other illnesses; the peak incidence is in the sixth decade and it is more common in men. It is radiographically characterized by gross colonic dilatation, scant air-fluid levels, gradual transition to a collapsed bowel, and a normal gas and fecal pattern in the rectum.[9] Treatment is increasingly focusing on the use of mechanical measures (usually endoscopic) for decompression.[8]

Chronic pseudo-obstruction is an uncommon syndrome characterized by symptoms and signs of intestinal obstruction in the absence of a mechanical blockage. It is associated with nausea, vomiting, abdominal distention, abdominal pain, and constipation. The pathophysiology of chronic pseudo-obstruction is best understood in the context of either a myopathy (including scleroderma, amyloidosis, and hollow visceral myopathy) or a neuropathy. Postural dizziness, visual disturbances, and sweating abnormalities suggest an autonomic neuropathy, whereas urinary symptoms suggest genitourinary involvement by a generalized visceral neuromyopathic disorder.

In searching for the cause of chronic pseudo-obstruction, the clinician should inquire about use of anticholinergic agents, phenothiazines, antihypertensive agents such as clonidine, and tricyclic antidepressants. Identification of a neuropathic basis may require an extensive search for underlying factors, such as a brain tumor. Structural examination with computed tomographic scanning or magnetic resonance imaging and noninvasive tests of autonomic function are indicated to detect a treatable lesion. Myopathic and neuropathic disorders can be distinguished by small bowel manometry[8]; myopathies are characterized by low pressure waves, neuropathies by uncoordinated waves of normal amplitude. Disorders of the enteric (intrinsic) nervous system should be suspected when manometrically confirmed chronic intestinal pseudo-obstruction is not associated with a demonstrable lesion in the extrinsic neural supply (Fig 1).[8]

Small Bowel Motility Disorders

The spectrum of clinical syndromes involving small bowel dysmotility is broad, ranging from stasis syndromes after abdominal surgery to myopathic

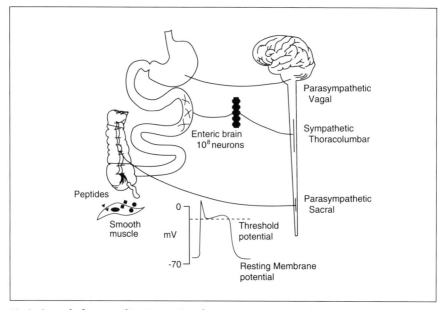

Fig 1. Control of gut motility. Interactions between extrinsic neural pathways and the intrinsic nervous system ("enteric brain") modulate contractions of gastrointestinal smooth muscle. Peptide-receptor interactions alter muscle membrane potentials by stimulating bidirectional ion fluxes. In turn, membrane characteristics dictate whether or not the muscle cell contracts.

and neuropathic disorders. The pathophysiology of abnormal small bowel motility can usually be attributed to a myopathic or a neuropathic disorder.[8] Basal manometry can help distinguish between neuropathic and myopathic disorders and indicate which patients are likely to respond to therapy. When the smooth muscle is destroyed, currently available pharmacologic agents cannot be expected to help.[8]

Postoperative Disorders
Disturbances of proximal bowel motility are frequently observed in patients after gastric surgery. We recently studied 60 patients who had been referred for manometry because of stasis after gastric surgery.[10] Nausea, vomiting, bloating, abdominal pain, and weight loss were the most common symptoms. Two thirds of the patients had a well-documented history of peptic ulcer before surgery. Twelve patients had undergone truncal vagotomy and a "drainage operation," and the other 48 had a partial gastrectomy with a gastroenterostomy (either Billroth I, Billroth II, or Roux-en-Y). Clearly, vagotomy or surgical disruption of enteric continuity could aggravate or uncover preexisting abnormal motor function.

Chronic gastric atony occasionally may occur as a complication of truncal vagotomy. Atony is a disabling condition characterized by pain, nausea, and vomiting and may also be a complication of diabetes mellitus. Medical treatment is often disappointing and additional resective surgery may be needed. Karlstrom and Kelly[11] followed 39 patients after treatment of postsurgical gastroparesis by extensive subtotal or near-total gastrectomy and Roux-en-Y gastrojejunostomy. They found that 79% of patients had fewer symptoms postoperatively than preoperatively. This approach might be considered radical, but nearly all the patients had failed lesser gastric revision operations, and all were long-term gastric cripples.[11]

Myopathic Disorders

A group of generalized disorders of smooth muscle or a condition that targets hollow organs such as the gut and urinary tract can also affect the small bowel and predispose a patient to dysmotility. These disorders include the following:

- **Amyloidosis.** Amyloidosis infiltrates muscle layers. Manometry may be able to differentiate it from amyloid neuropathy.
- **Systemic sclerosis.** Frequently associated with symptoms of gastrointestinal motor dysfunction, systemic sclerosis (scleroderma) is believed to originate with a neuropathic process. This is followed by infiltration of the muscle layers with fibrous tissue, resulting in myopathy. Manifestations of this disorder have been confirmed in the stomach and small bowel.[12]
- **Dermatomyositis.** Gut motor disturbance is a well-recognized, though rare, feature of dermatomyositosis.[13] Abnormalities of gut smooth muscle may be associated with weakness of skeletal muscle, resulting in impaired upper gut propulsion.
- **Dystrophia myotonica.** This disorder impairs muscle function at virtually all levels of the gastrointestinal tract. Degenerative changes in smooth muscles of the small intestine and colon, with fatty infiltration and collagen formation among smooth muscle cells, are similar to changes observed in dystrophic skeletal muscle.[14]
- **Hollow visceral myopathy.** Impaired gastrointestinal motor function related to this disorder occurs in a broad spectrum of patients. Occasionally, only asymptomatic duodenal involvement may be present. Contrast x-ray examination of the gut demonstrates dilatation and hypocontractility, and manometric studies show low pressure of contractions in the affected regions.[8]

Neuropathic Disorders

Diseases of extrinsic neural control or of the enteric nervous system are also associated with disorders of small bowel motility. These neuropathies may be acute or chronic. In acute peripheral neuropathy, autonomic dysfunction associated with certain acute viral infections may result in nausea, vomiting, abdominal cramps, constipation, or an illness compatible with pseudo obstruction. Guillian-Barre syndrome, herpes varicella zoster, and Epstein-Barr virus are infections that may cause persistent gastrointestinal motor disturbances.

Among the disorders of diabetes mellitus and amyloidosis are the most common causes of gastrointestinal motor dysfunction. The effects of diabetic autonomic neuropathy on the gut are well known and gastrointestinal symptoms are common in diabetic patients. Additional neuropathies associated with disorders of small intestinal motility include pandysautonomia, idiopathic orthostatic hypotension, spinal cord injury, and brain disease. Patients with Parkinson's disease, for example, are known to have delayed gastric emptying aggravated by treatment with levodopa.[15]

Functional Disorders

Nonulcer Dyspepsia

Poorly defined and widely misunderstood, dyspepsia presents with few symptoms that allow physicians to characterize it. Best defined as chronic or recurrent upper abdominal pain or nausea, dyspepsia without an ulcer is diagnosed twice as often as is peptic ulceration. Patients with nonulcer dyspepsia have symptoms that prompt the physician to believe an ulcer may be present, but no ulcer is found on evaluation. Among disorders that need to be excluded in patients with symptoms of nonulcer dyspepsia are peptic ulcer disease, gastroesophageal reflux, aerophagia, cholelithiasis, chronic pancreatitis, and irritable bowel syndrome.[16] The priority is to rule out peptic ulceration. Although clinical features may help, endoscopic examination of the stomach and duodenum is necessary to rule out peptic ulcer and to diagnose nonulcer dyspepsia. Endoscopy provides a sensitivity of 92% and specificity of 100%.[17,18]

However, not all patients with dyspepsia can or should undergo endoscopy immediately, recommends the Health and Public Policy Committee of the American College of Physicians.[19] The committee suggests that endoscopy should be reserved only for dyspeptic patients refractory to symptomatic therapy with either antacids or H_2 receptor blockers. The yield from early endoscopy is only 30% in patients younger than 40 years of age but nearly 60% in patients older than 65. Early endoscopy appears merited especially in patients older than 40 with the onset of dyspepsia, chronic symptoms that have not previously been investigated, or clinical features suggestive of organic disease. In those under age 40 who have no evidence of organic disease or family history of peptic ulceration, it may be sufficient to counsel the patient and offer reassurance. If patients in this subset fail to show improvement after 7 to 10 days, during which they have followed advice not to smoke or consume alcohol and have received an antacid, endoscopy is appropriate. If symptoms have not completely resolved within 6 to 8 weeks, endoscopy is recommended to exclude peptic ulcer and gastric cancer (Fig 2).[20–22]

Irritable Bowel Syndrome

Irritable bowel syndrome is a symptom complex that is thought to involve mainly the lower bowel. Abdominal pain, alteration of bowel function (closely related to the pain), and bloating are the cardinal features. Nausea and vomiting may occur but usually are not dominant symptoms.

Psychogenic Causes

Psychopathology is often a fellow traveler with motility disorders and may even be involved directly as a cause of nausea and vomiting. In patients at high risk for an eating disorder with a psychogenic basis—namely, bulimia and anorexia nervosa—nausea and vomiting in the presence of other signs consistent with the suspected diagnosis may signify the need for a psychiatric referral.

Although psychologic traits appear to be unrelated to the development of gastrointestinal motility disorders per se, psychologic symptoms do influence whether a patient consults a physician.[5] Everyday stresses may, independently of psychopathology, alter gastrointestinal motility and produce bowel symptoms.

The extent to which psychiatric disorders play a role in altering gastrointestinal motility is still controversial. The consensus seems to be that there is an excess of psychopathology in patients with gastrointestinal motility disorders, but no specific psychiatric condition is strongly associated with disturbance of motility. Depression and anxiety, the most common disorders associated with motility problems, are also the most common diagnoses in the general population.[5]

Diagnostic Evaluation

Investigations

Assuming a history and physical examination have not provided suggestive diagnostic clues concerning a psychiatric basis to the unexplained nausea and vomiting, and a gastrointestinal cause is suspected based on the initial assessment, more sophisticated testing is needed (Fig 3).

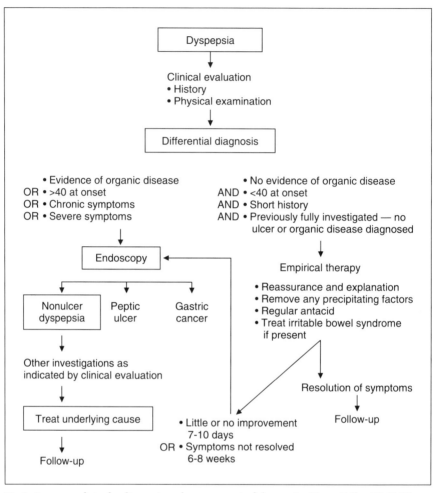

Fig 2. An approach to the diagnosis and management of dyspepsia. (From Talley NJ, Phillips SF. Non-ulcer dyspepsia: potential causes and pathophysiology. *Ann Intern Med.* **1991;108:865–879.)**

It has been argued that the characteristics of a patient's symptoms can be overemphasized.[1] For example, the timing of vomiting in relation to meals, the presence or absence of nausea, and descriptions such as projectile vomiting or retention-type vomiting may be misleading.[1] Patients with motility disorders may have fasting nausea and vomiting either exclusively or in combination with postprandial vomiting[1] (Fig 4).

A priority in the initial phase of the work-up is to determine whether the patient's condition is acute or chronic. Acute symptoms (<24 hours) often represent a component of the systemic response to a painful visceral

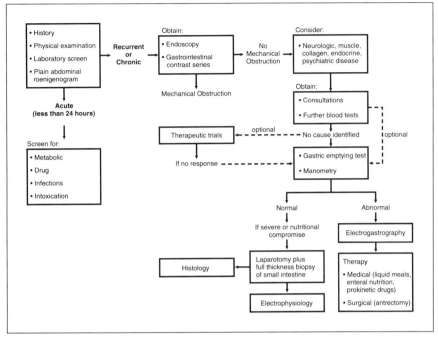

Fig 3. Algorithm for management of patients with unexplained vomiting. (From Malagelada J-R, Camilleri M. Unexplained vomiting: a diagnostic challenge. *Ann Intern Med.* 1984;101:211–218.)

lesion (reflex vomiting), drug reaction or intoxication, or metabolic disorder. Recurrent nausea and vomiting will likely require more extensive investigation, including radiologic studies and endoscopy of the upper gastrointestinal tract.

Conventional x-rays may demonstrate the lesion causing nausea and vomiting or provide indirect evidence of obstruction or motility disturbance (such as gastric dilatation, retained food and secretions, slow emptying of barium, or intestinal dilatation with slow transit).

Although it may be more sensitive and specific than radiologic studies in demonstrating upper gastrointestinal lesions, endoscopy is less useful in evaluating motor function, except to indicate the presence of retained food after an overnight fast.

In nonulcer dyspepsia, endoscopy is the gold standard. However, x-rays and endoscopy generally are valuable only to demonstrate mucosal or obstructive disease, because these examinations may be normal despite the presence of severe motility disorders.

Even a detailed history, careful physical examination, laboratory workup, barium contrast studies, x-ray evaluations, and endoscopy may fail to

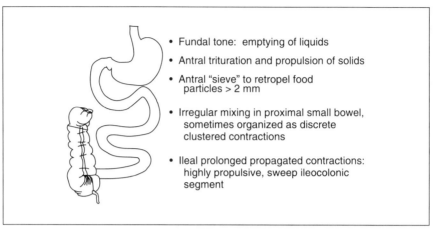

• Fundal tone: emptying of liquids

• Antral trituration and propulsion of solids

• Antral "sieve" to retropel food
  particles > 2 mm

• Irregular mixing in proximal small bowel,
  sometimes organized as discrete
  clustered contractions

• Ileal prolonged propagated contractions:
  highly propulsive, sweep ileocolonic
  segment

Fig 4. Major characteristics of postprandial gastrointestinal motility. (From Camilleri M, Phillips SF. Acute chronic intestinal pseudoobstruction. In: Stollerman GH, ed. *Advances in Internal Medicine*. St. Louis, Mo.: Mosby Year Book; 1991:287–306.)

provide evidence of a motility disorder. The decision to move to the next level of testing, however, is generally postponed. At this point, a therapeutic trial of a prokinetic agent (metoclopramide, domperidone, or bethanechol) or, when indicated clinically, antidepressant therapy, should be tried.

Patients who remain refractory to such therapy and in whom psychogenic vomiting is not suspected clinically should undergo further evaluation, with gastric emptying studies and manometry. Despite technical problems such as stability of isotope labelling, measurement of isotope counts, patient positioning, and interpretation of emptying curves, this may be the only way to objectively diagnose delayed gastric emptying and a gastric motility disturbance.[5] Whereas measurement of the rate of gastric emptying can confirm a clinical problem and help establish the presence of gastric stasis, emptying studies give no information about etiology. Esophageal manometry may be useful in establishing the cause of recurrent vomiting, because patients with gastrointestinal motor disorders may have clinically silent esophageal motor abnormalities.[1]

Possible Links Among These Conditions
Disordered motility of the upper gastrointestinal tract, suggested by abdominal distention, flatulence, and fullness after meals, may be a component of the nonulcer dyspepsia syndrome. Some evidence supporting an association between postprandial antral hypomotility and dyspepsia emerged from one manometric study; about half of the patients had gastric and intestinal abnormalities.[22] The issue is clouded, however, because many patients had associated metabolic and neurologic diseases, and symptoms were not well correlated with manometric results. In other studies of

patients with unexplained nausea and vomiting, abnormal myoelectric activity of the gastric muscle has been reported.[23-25] Overall, it is still unclear how these findings and symptoms are related.

Despite the lack of compelling evidence supporting a relationship between a motility disorder and dyspepsia, the possibility of such an association has led to treatment of these conditions with dopaminergic blockers, because dopamine inhibits gastric motility. Another theory suggests that functional disturbances of the upper gastrointestinal tract may be mediated hormonally. However, no strong associations have been established between motility disturbances, circulating concentrations of gut hormones, and symptoms of nonulcer dyspepsia.[18]

Intestinal pseudo-obstruction. The signs and symptoms of the disorder may initially resemble nonulcer dyspepsia, irritable bowel syndrome, or chronic idiopathic constipation.

Until more specific and less invasive techniques are developed, manometry is the key diagnostic test for chronic intestinal pseudo-obstruction, after x-ray examinations and endoscopy have excluded mechanical obstruction. Unless manometry is performed, frequent complaints of significant abdominal pain in patients with chronic pseudo-obstruction may lead to unnecessary laparotomy.[8] Small-bowel manometric studies may confirm a motility disorder; these abnormalities include aberrant configuration or propagation of phase III of the interdigestive migrating motor complex; sustained, uncoordinated pressure activity; intense bursts of phasic pressure activity; and failure of a meal to induce a fed pattern or to interrupt cyclic interdigestive motor activity. Should such patients ever need an abdominal operation, full-thickness biopsies of the areas involved with disease should be obtained.

Treatment

Impaired gastric emptying. The poor correlation between the results of gastric emptying studies and symptoms of gastroparesis has led to the recommendation that all symptomatic patients should be treated.[5] Prokinetic agents should be administered so that peak plasma levels are attained before meals, usually at least a half hour before eating.[5] An evening dose is important to normalize, as much as possible, the interdigestive myoelectric complex, which enables undigested material to empty from the stomach and minimizes bezoar formation.

The dopamine antagonist *domperidone* is sometimes useful, as is the benzamide *metoclopramide*; a third agent, *cisapride,* promotes the release of acetylcholine at the mysenteric plexus. Intravenous metoclopramide increases gastric emptying in diabetic and postvagotomy gastroparesis.[5] In contrast to metoclopramide, domperidone does not cross the blood-brain barrier, and it produces fewer side effects.[5] The most potent of the three prokinetic agents is cisapride, which acts more broadly on the gastrointestinal tract: it increases lower esophageal sphincter pressure, stimulates peristalsis in the esophagus and small bowel, and hastens gastric and duodenal emptying.[5]

Chronic gastroparesis and/or pseudo-obstruction. The goals of therapy are to maintain adequate nutrition and restore normal intestinal propulsion. Nutritional support varies with the severity of the problem but includes a low-lactose, low-fiber, polypeptide or hydrolyzed protein diet with multivitamins and supplementation with iron, folate, and calcium. Central parenteral nutrition is often required in severe cases. The potential for significant morbidity and mortality associated with central parenteral nutrition must be accepted in view of the extremely poor prognosis in severe forms of chronic intestinal pseudo-obstruction. Dietary and medical treatment are generally ineffective, and only a few patients are surgical candidates.[8]

Conclusion

The challenge of diagnosing a gastrointestinal motility disorder as the cause of unexplained nausea and vomiting lies in excluding a broad spectrum of illnesses, particularly those that are obstructive or psychogenic. If psychogenic, metabolic, and endocrine causes have been ruled out, the evaluation can focus on esophageal motility disorders, gastric motor function, and small bowel dysmotility. Radiographic and endoscopic studies are essential, but they may not provide compelling evidence of pathophysiology; in that case, more sophisticated and extensive testing, including the use of manometry and scintigraphic evaluation, may be required.

The aims of treatment are the correction of dehydration and malnutrition and the restoration of intestinal peristalsis for small bowel motility disorders. In mild cases, no specific treatment may be needed other than reassurance and control of symptoms. Pharmacologic agents such as bethanechol and metoclopramide have been disappointing, and the initial promise shown by cisapride and domperidone needs to be confirmed in larger trials of longer duration.

References

1. Malagelada J-R, Camilleri M. Unexplained vomiting: a diagnostic challenge. *Ann Intern Med.* 1984;101:211–218.
2. Johnson LF. 24-Hour pH monitoring in the study of gastroesophageal reflux. *J Clin Gastroenterol.* 1980;2:387–399.
3. Holzl R, Whitehead WE. *Psychophysiology of the Gastrointestinal Tract: Experimental and Clinical Applications.* New York, NY: Plenum Press; 1983.

4. Swanson DW, Swenson WM, Huizenga KA, et al. Persistent nausea without organic cause. *Mayo Clin Proc.* 1976;51:257–262.

5. Champion MC, ed. *Physiology, Diagnosis & Therapy in GI Motility Disorders.* Philadelphia, Pa: Medical Publishing Foundation; 1987.

6. Greenberger NJ, ed. *Gastrointestinal Disorders: A Pathophysiologic Approach.* Chicago, Ill: Year Book Medical Publishers; 1989.

7. Oh JJ, Kim CH. Gastroparesis after a presumed viral illness: clinical and laboratory features and natural history. *Mayo Clin Proc.* 1990;65:636–642.

8. Camilleri M, Phillips SF. Acute and chronic intestinal pseudoobstruction. In: Stollerman GH, ed. *Advances in Internal Medicine.* St. Louis, Mo: Mosby Year Book; 1991:287–306.

9. Gilchrist AM, Mills JO, Russell. Acute large bowel pseudoobstruction. *Clin Radiol.* 1985;36:401–404.

10. Fich A, Neri M, Camilleri M, et al. Stasis syndromes following gastric surgery: clinical and motility features of 60 symptomatic patients. *J Clin Gastroenterol.* 1990;12:505–512.

11. Karlstrom L, Kelly KA. Roux-Y gastrectomy for chronic gastric atony. *Am J Surgery.* 1989;157:44–49.

12. Greydanus M, Camilleri M. Abnormal postcibal antral and small bowel motility in systemic sclerosis. *Gastroenterology.* 1989;96:110–115.

13. Feldman F, Marshak RH. Dermatomyositis with significant involvement of the gastrointestinal tract. *Am J Roentgenol.* 1963;90:746.

14. Nowak TV, Anuras S, Brown BP. Small intestinal motility in myotonic dystrophy patients. *Gastroenterology.* 1984;86:808.

15. Evans MA, Broe GA, Triggs EJ. Gastric emptying rate and the systemic availability of levodopa in the elderly parkinsonian patient. *Neurology.* 1981;31:1288.

16. Talley NJ, Phillips SF. Non-ulcer dyspepsia: potential causes and pathophysiology. *Ann Intern Med.* 108:865–879.

17. Brown P, Salmon PR, Burwood RG, et al. The endoscopic, radiological, and surgical findings in chronic duodenal ulceration. *Scand J Gastroenterol.* 1978;13:557–560.

18. Colin-Jones DG. Endoscopy or radiology for upper gastrointestinal symptoms. *Lancet.* 1986;1:1022–1023.

19. Health and Public Policy Committee, American College of Physicians. Endoscopy in the evaluation of dyspepsia. *Ann Intern Med.* 1985;102:266–269.

20. Sampliner RE. Are H2 blockers for symptom relief? *J Clin Gastroenterol.* 1986;8:8–9. Editorial.

21. Kahn KL, Greenfield S. The efficacy of endoscopy in the evaluation of dyspepsia: a review of the literature and development of a sound strategy. *J Clin Gastroenterol.* 1986;8:346–358.

22. Malagelada JR, Stanghellini V. Manometric evaluation of functional upper gut symptoms. *Gastroenterology.* 1985;88:1223–1231.

23. You CH, Chey WY. Study of electromechanical activity of the stomach in humans and in dogs with particular attention to tachygastria. *Gastroenterology.* 1984;86:1460–1468.

24. Chey WY, You CH, Lee KY, et al. Gastric dysrhythmia: clinical aspects. In: Chey WY, ed. *Functional Disorders of the Digestive Tract.* New York, NY: Raven Press; 1983:175–181.

25. Geldof H, Van Der Schee EJ, Van Blankenstein M, et al. Electrogastrographic study of gastric myoelectrical activity in patients with unexplained nausea and vomiting. *Gut.* 1986;27:799–808.

Nausea and Vomiting Complicating Pregnancy

Tekoa King, CNM, MPH, and Julian T. Parer, MD, PhD

Occurring with such frequency that they are considered almost diagnostic of pregnancy, nausea and vomiting are perhaps the most troublesome symptoms of gestation. These discomforts accompany about half of all pregnancies and usually disappear by the end of the first trimester.[1] Nausea of pregnancy is usually most apparent in the morning and wanes during the day.

Nausea and vomiting of pregnancy were described as early as 2000 BC, but despite a multitude of studies since, the precise etiologic mechanisms are still unknown. Numerous theories for the underlying cause of this disorder have given rise to a broad spectrum of treatments. The most important issue for clinicians is whether symptoms are serious and persistent enough to warrant the diagnosis hyperemesis, a disorder characterized by pernicious vomiting and associated with potentially life-threatening sequelae.

Although the term *nausea and vomiting of pregnancy* is applicable to both mild and severe forms, its use should be restricted to the syndrome commonly observed during the first 14 to 16 weeks, which is characterized by some disturbance in appetite.[2] Normal symptoms vary from morning nausea to occasional vomiting; signs of disturbed nutritional balance are absent. In contrast, the terms *hyperemesis gravidarum* or *pernicious vomiting of pregnancy* best describe the condition that occurs in a small number of patients who develop intractable vomiting and disturbed nutrition, such as alteration of electrolyte balance, weight loss of 5% or more, ketosis, and acetonuria. Hyperemesis, if unresolved, can ultimately lead to retinal hemorrhage, liver and kidney damage, and neurologic disturbances.[2]

A profile of the woman at risk for nausea and vomiting of pregnancy has emerged from epidemiologic studies. Researchers from the National Institute of Health (NIH) reviewed 9098 pregnancies from the Collaborative Perinatal Project database and found nausea and vomiting (not hyperemesis or gastroenteritis) in 56% of these pregnancies.[3] These researchers found nausea and vomiting to be more common among the following groups:

- Primigravidas
- Young women (the incidence is highest among woman younger than 20 years old and drops significantly after age 35)
- Women with fewer than 12 years of education
- Women with a history of nausea and vomiting in an earlier pregnancy. Women who have nausea and vomiting in one pregnancy are more likely to vomit in subsequent pregnancies when compared with women who did not have the syndrome in an earlier pregnancy.[3]
- Women weighing 77.1 kg (170 lbs) or more

Paradoxically, the NIH researchers and other researchers have found that the presence of nausea and vomiting is associated with a favorable pregnancy outcome. Women reporting vomiting were less likely to experience miscarriage or stillbirth. Interestingly, no differences were found in infant birth weight between mothers who did and who did not experience vomiting.

Etiology

Despite substantial investigation, the etiology of nausea and vomiting remains obscure.[4] The concept of a multifactorial basis to nausea and vomiting in pregnancy is gaining wider acceptance.

The absence of structural disease within the gastrointestinal tract suggests the possibility of disordered upper gastrointestinal motility, akin to that seen after some viral infections, total body radiation, diabetic gastroparesis, and a range of diseases that can cause the syndrome of intestinal pseudo-obstruction.[4]

Other etiologic theories focus on a hormonal stimulus. The hormonal changes that may underlie nausea and vomiting include high levels of circulating estrogen and human chorionic gonadotropin (hCG).[5] It is postulated that these agents may directly stimulate the chemoreceptor cells in the postrema of the medulla, adjacent to the point where the emetic response is believed to be coordinated.

Evidence of a relationship between vomiting and hCG was also apparent in a Japanese study. Emesis usually occurs in the first trimester, when cg levels are high. In this cohort, the mean level of hCG was highest in the group with nausea and vomiting and intermediate in the group that was nauseated only[6] (Fig 1). This study confirmed previous findings of higher serum hCG levels in patients with emesis compared with asymptomatic women.[7]

The connection between hCG and hyperthyroidism is well known, as hCG has a thyroid-stimulating effect.[8] Biochemical or clinical hyperthy-

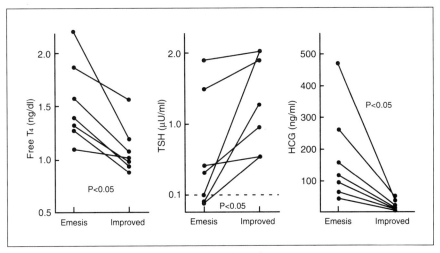

Fig 1. Serum levels of free thyroxine (T_4), thyroid-stimulating hormone (TSH), and human chorionic gonadotiopin (hCG) at the time of emesis and after improvement in seven pregnant women. (From Mor M, et al. Morning sickness and thyroid function in normal pregnancy. *Obstet Gynecol.* 1988;72:355–359.)

roidism is often observed in patients with hydatidiform mole or choriocarcinoma (i.e., in patients with high levels of circulating hCG).[9] According to the Japanese authors,[6] the significant correlation they found between serum concentrations of hCG and free thyroxine (T_4) strongly suggests that the thyroid gland is physiologically activated in early pregnancy by hCG or a related substance, which may also induce gestational emesis.

The above observations led the Japanese researchers to investigate a further relationship between morning sickness and thyroid function.[6] These researchers found a significant increase in serum free T_4 and a decrease in serum thyroid-stimulating hormone (TSH) in early pregnancy. These changes were especially marked in subjects with nausea and vomiting. The authors suggest that when an increased serum free T_4 level is detected in a pregnant woman, her thyroid should be carefully palpated. Serum levels of antithyroid microsomal antibody and thyroid-stimulating antibody should be measured to differentiate Graves' disease; however, the increase in thyroid-stimulating antibody is low in early pregnancy even in patients with thyrotoxic Graves' disease.[6]

Controversy surrounds the role of psychologic stress in inducing nausea and vomiting during pregnancy. A 1988 study in Greece of 102 women in the first trimester suggests that psychologic factors must be implicated in at least a small number of cases.[10] Iatrakis et al[10] proposed that feelings of insecurity arising from poor communication with the husband and stress, doubts, or inadequate information about pregnancy and the health of the fetus may lead to subconscious resentment and the figurative rejection of pregnancy, symbolized by vomiting. The Greek researchers found that during the first 12 weeks of pregnancy, vomiting and nausea were positively correlated with an unsuitable diet, large and infrequent meals, and poor communication with the husband and the obstetrician.[10]

Management of Mild Nausea and Vomiting

The cornerstone of initial treatment for nausea and vomiting remains non-pharmacologic. Although supported only by anecdotal evidence, common recommendations are small, frequent meals; dry crackers upon rising (to minimize the emptiness of the stomach); avoidance of strong odors, spicy foods, and cold liquids.[5] Other suggestions include ingestion of sweet foods before bedtime or upon rising, restriction of dietary fats, and avoidance of fluids and solids together. Reassurance, however, is perhaps the most effective remedy for typical cases of mild morning sickness, as the condition usually resolves by the sixteenth week of pregnancy.

Occasionally, the problem is refractory to these relatively simple approaches. Drug therapy can be considered if nausea and vomiting significantly interfere with the patient's ability to perform normal daily activities, or if objective signs, such as weight loss or urinary ketosis, are evident. Approximately 10% of women require medication for mild nausea and vomiting.

Pyridoxine (vitamin B_6), a water-soluble B complex vitamin that is an essential coenzyme in the metabolism of amino acids, carbohydrates, and lipids, has been shown to be effective in selected patients. In the one randomized placebo-controlled study done to date at the University of Iowa, 31 women received vitamin B_6, 25 mg orally every 8 hours for 72 hours, and 28 women received placebo. Pyridoxine did not improve symptoms in patients with mild to moderate nausea, but it significantly reduced vomiting in pregnant women complaining of severe nausea. After completing therapy, only 8 of the 31 patients given the active treatment had any vomiting, compared with 15 of the 28 control patients.[11] Used as early as 1942, vitamin B_6 was included in the formulation of Bendectin. This agent was used to treat nausea and vomiting of pregnancy until 1983, when the manufacturer removed it from the market in the face of litigation claiming the drug caused congenital malformations. (See below.)

The requirements for vitamin B_6 are increased during pregnancy, but low serum concentrations generally are not found until the second and third trimesters.[12] Pyridoxine deficiency is not evidenced clinically, and a relationship is seen between vitamin B_6 levels and the incidence or degree of morning sickness in pregnant women.

Because nausea and vomiting during pregnancy tend to be self-limited and often respond to measures such as small, frequent meals, most women can be managed without the use of therapeutic agents, which are best reserved for severe cases.

Hyperemesis

In contrast to emesis gravidarum, the transitory morning sickness occurring in at least half of normal gestations, hyperemesis gravidarum or intractable gestational vomiting is a more pernicious syndrome of the first trimester, occurring in approximately 3 of 1,000 pregnancies.[13] Characterized by weight loss, electrolyte imbalance, and disturbed nutrition, hyperemesis frequently requires admission to the hospital. The clinical course is extremely variable, with the greatest likelihood for hospital admission between the eighth and twelfth weeks.[1]

Hyperemesis frequently begins in the morning, and its initial symptoms resemble those of classic morning sickness. The vomiting becomes increasingly frequent and may be unremitting in advanced cases. In severe cases, tachycardia, oliguria, a rising urinary specific gravity, and progressive ketosis develop.[13] As the condition worsens, hemoconcentration becomes evident, the blood urea nitrogen level is elevated, and serum sodium, chloride, and potassium concentrations decline. Replacement of fluid and electrolytes can eliminate the severe complications and risk of mortality associated with hyperemesis. Vitamin replacement and carbohydrate supplementation, with or without central hyperalimentation, have also contributed to improved prognosis for pregnant women with hyperemesis.

Differential Diagnosis
The crucial task for the clinician is differentiating between normal nausea and vomiting of gestation (emesis gravidarum) and the pernicious form of vomiting (hyperemesis gravidarum). The distinction is complicated because it is one of degree only[13]; clinically, no sharp demarcation between the two conditions is evident. Most authors apply the term hyperemesis gravidarum to patients requiring hospitalization.[13] The criteria for hospital admission are not standardized and may depend on economic factors, clinical course, and the response to medications and other outpatient therapy. Timing of symptoms is important: true hyperemesis is a condition restricted to the first trimester.[13] Only in rare cases does it continue beyond 12 to 14 weeks. If symptoms do persist beyond this period, they usually are

not of the same intensity. Vomiting that begins late in the second or third trimester usually signifies some other disorder.

A wide range of other disorders—including gastrointestinal and endocrine abnormalities—could masquerade as hyperemesis, as their initial presentation also may be nausea and vomiting. Primary parathyroidism, for example, may produce a clinical picture indistinguishable from hyperemesis. This disorder can be correctly diagnosed by an elevated serum calcium level (>15 mg/dL), accompanied by depressed concentrations of magnesium and phosphorus in a patient with acute symptoms. Management relies on normalizing calcium levels, restoring vascular volume, and replenishing potassium and magnesium. Hyperemesis also should be differentiated from conditions such as appendicitis and pyelonephritis.[14] These disorders must be excluded before the diagnosis of hyperemesis can be confirmed.[13]

Risk Factors

Pinpointing risk factors for hyperemesis is difficult, because studies tend to differ on which historical and demographic features are most important. Those most commonly mentioned, include:

(1) previous history of hyperemesis
(2) multiple pregnancy
(3) first pregnancy (Fig 2)
(4) young maternal age (Fig 2)

A prior history of hyperemesis is the most important factor.[13] Recurrence rates range from 26% to 50%. It is less clear whether multiple pregnancy increases the likelihood of hyperemesis.[1] Proponents of the theory that high levels of hCG have an etiologic role in the condition cite the higher incidence of hyperemesis in twin pregnancy as further proof of their case. While the role of multiple pregnancy is controversial, the consensus is that hyperemesis is more common when additional fetuses are present.[13] The influence of parity is also controversial: studies in Caucasian populations have detected an increased incidence of hyperemesis in the first pregnancy,[3,15] while studies in non-Caucasian populations have failed to find significant differences between the first and later gestations.

Cigarette smoking appears to have a negative correlation with hyperemesis. Investigators have speculated that the protective effect may be related to depressed estrogen levels in women who smoke.[13]

Etiology

Association with hCG serum levels. Mounting evidence suggests an association between hyperemesis and the serum concentration of hCG, but the data are not conclusive. The disappearance of hyperemesis at the

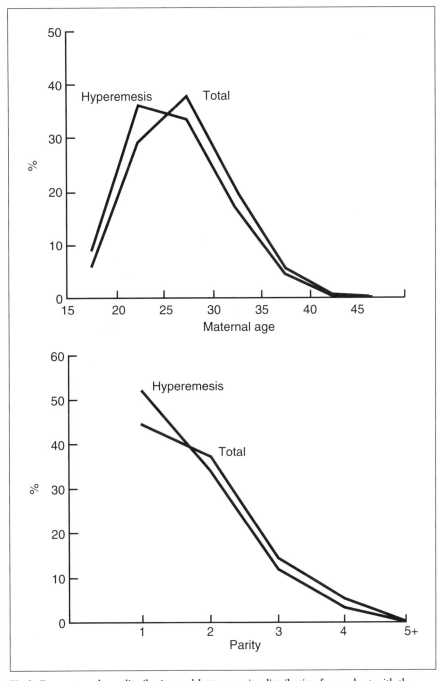

Fig 2. *Top*, maternal age distribution and *bottom*, parity distribution for a cohort with the diagnosis of hyperemesis and for the total population. (From Kallen B. Hyperemesis during pregnancy and delivery outcome: a registry study. *Eur J Obstet Gynecol Reprod Biol.* 1987;26:291–302.)

end of the first trimester closely parallels the physiologic decline of hCG, and many observers have noted the association between peak incidence of emesis and maximum maternal serum hCG levels.[1] The use of hCG immunoassays has produced more data to address this issue, but the controversy is far from settled because the assay technique, patient populations, and timing of sampling vary. Because hydration, ambulation, and the sex of the fetus affect hCG levels, they may also be factors to consider in determining the validity of the hCG hypothesis. Nevertheless, the association between serum concentrations of hCG and the nausea and vomiting of pregnancy is one of the strongest explanations offered for the pathophysiology of hyperemesis gravidarum.

The thyroid connection. It is important to investigate thyroid function in patients with hyperemesis for several reasons. Although rare, frank hyperthyroidism or classic Graves' disease increases the risk of poor outcomes, including intrauterine growth retardation, and maternal complications such as delirium, hypertension, convulsions, and high-output cardiac failure.[16] In addition, the symptoms of thyrotoxicosis may masquerade as those of hyperemesis and the two conditions can be confused easily. Further, 40% to 70% of women hospitalized with hyperemesis also have abnormalities of thyroid function.[13]

Patients presumed to have hyperemesis should be screened for thyroid function (eg, TSH, T_4, T_3, free T_4, and thyroid index). Results of tests for TSH receptor antibodies separate patients with hyperemesis and "physiologic" thyroid dysfunction from those with thyrotoxicosis, as only patients with Graves' disease have these antibodies.[13] If thyrotoxicosis is confirmed, standard antithyroid treatment is indicated. In general, abnormalities of thyroid function in patients with hyperemesis are short-lived and self-limited, requiring no treatment.

The role of estrogen. Although its association with hyperemesis has not been explored as extensively as the connection with hCG, elevated estrogen levels could be another factor in the etiology of hyperemesis. This intriguing possibility was first considered after a 1987 study observed an elevated risk for testicular cancer in the sons of women who had hyperemesis during pregnancy.[17] Corroborating evidence is the fact that, like hCG concentrations, levels of estradiol also increase rapidly in pregnant women who experience morning sickness.

Measuring hormones in the first trimester in 35 women with hyperemesis and 35 control women matched for age, parity, and medical center, a California study[17] found that mean levels of total estradiol were 26% higher and mean levels of sex-hormone binding-globulin binding capacity were 37% higher in patients with hyperemesis than in control subjects. In contrast, the differences in hCG concentrations between the two groups were not statistically significant, tending to downplay the importance of the hCG theory. This study suggested that an extremely rapid rise in estradiol level is the likely cause of vomiting, especially if sex-hormone binding–globulin binding accelerates after a delay following the rise in estradiol.[17] In support of this theory is the observation that nausea often occurs when estrogens are administered clinically and subsides when estrogens are withdrawn.

Psychogenic factors. A century ago, psychologic factors were thought to be the primary cause of hyperemesis. Early psychoanalytic reports offered the oversimplified notion that vomiting is a symbolic rejection of pregnancy, an unconscious attempt to reject the child. This concept gave rise to punitive approaches to treatment, including prolonged hospitalization, denial of visitors, and isolation of the patients. The presumed role of psychologic factors has begun to recede as studies emphasize the importance of an endocrinologic basis for hyperemesis, and the psychogenic viewpoint is now somewhat controversial.

Nevertheless, the psychiatric literature includes not only the older anecdotal case studies but also large, controlled studies with objective psychologic measures and specific psychiatric diagnostic criteria. Several psychiatric syndromes appear to be associated with hyperemesis, including the following:

- *Histrionic personality disorder;* characterized by overdramatization of symptoms, emotional lability, and self-centeredness.[18]
- *Borderline personality disorder;* typically manifested by chronic conflicts, unstable relationships, chronic depression, and self-destructive behavior.
- *Somatization disorder;* characterized by multiple medical complaints, starting early in life, that are incompletely explained by physical causes.[18]

Although elaborate attempts have been made to link hyperemesis directly with psychosomatic factors, the consensus favors a multifactorial etiology with interplay among a range of factors. One of the more popular views suggests that the underlying etiology of hyperemesis is primarily endocrinologic, but the clinical manifestations heavily depend on the individual's psychosocial characteristics.[13] Many women with hyperemesis experience overwhelming stress and have a history of vomiting under similar circumstances. Many others, however, have no psychiatric disorders and are helped by intravenous hydration and/or brief hospitalizations.[13]

Complications

Physicians have long assumed that nausea and vomiting predict a favorable outcome in pregnancy, but recent findings in patients with hyperemesis prompt reanalysis of this assumption. In the studies which have found that the presence of nausea and vomiting is favorably associated with normal fetal weight and decreased risk of spontaneous abortion, investigators have used varying definitions for the diagnosis of hyperemesis.[19] When stricter criteria are used and data from more clearly defined subsets of patients with hyperemesis are analyzed, it appears that hyperemesis adversely affects birth weight.

A well-designed Canadian study[19] challenged the long-standing belief that nausea and vomiting predict a good outcome. The study, based on a 5-year analysis at a Toronto hospital, found that the critical variable is loss of more than 5% of prepregnancy weight. The average birth weights of infants whose mothers met the criterion were significantly smaller for gestational age. Growth retardation (birth weight less than the 10th percentile) was also significantly more common in infants of women whose weight dropped more than 5%. Hypokalemia was found only in this group of patients, emphasizing the electrolyte disturbances associated with significant hyperemesis.[19] This study was unable to associate the presence of ketonuria with growth retardation, confirming previous suggestions of the common and nonspecific nature of ketonuria in pregnant women.[20] The Toronto study dramatizes the importance of early and aggressive treatment to prevent significant weight loss and enhance good perinatal outcomes.

While finding additional evidence of the adverse impact of hyperemesis on pregnancy outcomes, Chinese investigators[21] disagreed with the criterion of at least 5% weight loss. Claiming that the use of such weight loss is impractical because few women can recall their weights prior to pregnancy, these authors compared birth outcomes in 46 patients with severe hyperemesis and 26 with mild hyperemesis with outcomes of 8,802 deliveries in the same institution. Among the 46 patients with severe hyperemesis were 3 women who had preterm deliveries (less than 37 weeks gestation) and 9 who had babies with birth weights below the 10th percentile. Only one patient in the mild hyperemesis group had a low–birth weight baby, and none delivered preterm. These results imply that the metabolic disturbances created by persistent vomiting may create an adverse intrauterine environment that affects fetal growth.[21] Calling attention to their earlier findings of a higher incidence of hyperemesis in eclamptic pregnancies, the Chinese team advised that women with hyperemesis should be regarded as a high-risk group deserving close follow-up to detect development of pre-eclampsia and intrauterine growth retardation.[21]

Other disorders more often associated with alcoholism can appear in patients with hyperemesis.[13] Prolonged retching, for example, can result in rupture of the esophageal varices. In unusually severe or prolonged cases, Wernicke-Korsakoff encephalopathy, a syndrome caused by deficiency in vitamin B_1, may occur. A medical emergency, this syndrome should be managed immediately with administration of thiamine; the prognosis depends upon the speed with which the patient is treated.

Treatment

In contrast to the clinical course of mild episodes of morning sickness, which are usually self-limited and relatively easy to manage, hyperemesis poses several concerns for treatment. The weight loss, dehydration, and electrolyte abnormalities associated with the severe form of this disorder place the mother, and to a lesser degree the fetus, at risk.[13] Also, in cases with pathopsychologic components, outpatient medical therapy may not be effective, and such patients usually require hospitalization and psychosocial evaluations.[13]

Fairweather reported that the peak incidence of hospital admissions for hyperemesis is between the eight and twelfth week.[1] Little information is available on the length of hospital stay required. Generally, complete remission of symptoms occurs within 72 hours of intravenous replacement therapy. A frequent problem, however, is the patient who requires several readmissions because of recurrent symptoms. The best guide of satisfactory response to treatment and fitness for discharge is not simply cessation of vomiting, rehydration, and electrolyte balance, but also evidence of a steady gain in weight.[1] Those women who are discharged while the weight curve is still flat or falling, even though they are free from vomiting and apparently cured, are at high risk for readmission.

The cornerstone of treatment remains hospital admission, with fluid and electrolyte replacement and psychological support.[13] Correction of dehydration and normalization of blood chemistry are the primary and initial goals (Table 1). The following recommendations should help to restore hydration and normalize blood chemistry:

- Administer dextrose in a balanced salt solution, 3 L every 24 hours or more rapidly according to the extent of dehydration.[13]
- Provide supplemental potassium (60 mEq every 24 hours) by addition of concentrated KCl to the intravenous solution.
- Administer 100 mg or more of thiamine as well as 1 g of magnesium sulfate in the same solution every 24 hours if vomiting is severe and prolonged.

Table 1. Basic Treatment for Hyperemesis Gravidarum

1. Hospital admission for observation and vital sign recording.

2. Serial determinations of hemoglobin/hematocrit, renal function tests.

3. Daily weights, testing of urines for ketones and specific gravity. Calculation of intake and output.

4. Exclusion of specific medical conditions by appropriate evaluation; ie, urine culture, thyroid panel, liver function tests.

5. Intravenous therapy including magnesium and B vitamins to correct dehydration electrolyte imbalance and partially offset carbohydrate deficiencies; in unusual cases, central hyperalimentation.

6. Use of antiemetic agents, as required.

7. Psychological support, as necessary.

8. Abdominal or transvaginal ultrasonography to establish the gestational age and normality of pregnancy.

From O'Grady JP, Cohen LM. Emesis and hyperemesis gravidarum. In: O'Grady JP, Rosenthal M, eds. *Obstetrics: Psychological and Psychiatric Syndromes.* New York, NY: Elsevier; 1992.

Oral intake of foods should resume slowly after retching has resolved (i.e., after 24 hours without vomiting). Dietary supplements of iron and vitamins should be omitted until episodes of vomiting have ceased, as these products potentiate nausea.

The personal preferences of physicians for specific drugs have created a long list of medications commonly prescribed for hyperemesis. Such agents include chlorpromazine, dimenhydrinate, metoclopramide, and promethazine. The least toxic agent(s) should be administered in the lowest possible dose and for the shortest possible duration. Promethazine (50 mg per rectum every 4 to 6 hours) or prochlorperazine (10 mg intramuscularly or orally or 25 mg suppository every 6 hours) may be given acutely as antiemetics. However, withholding oral feeding and maintaining hydration intravenously are more effective in controlling vomiting.

For outpatient management, some patients with recurrent bouts of severe nausea may respond when rehydration is achieved either by an indwelling peripheral venous line (changed every 48 hours or as needed) or, in rare cases, by an indwelling major venous access line (Hickman catheter or similar device). To avoid hospitalization, Grady and Cohen[13] recommend that feeding be withheld while women with hyperemesis undergo intravenous therapy. Such patients should also either maintain close telephone contact with their physician or remain under the watchful supervision of a visiting nurse. Intravenous hyperalimentation may be required in prolonged or severe cases.[22]

Bendectin.   Used by 25% of all pregnant women in the late 1970s and early 1980s, Bendectin has left a large legacy of lawsuits regarding congenital malformations associated with its use. The teratogenicity of Bendectin doubtless will be debated for years. Although the drug has long been off the market, its antinausea ingredient is still available to clinicians in the drug Unisom. A sleeping aid, Unisom contains 25 mg of doxylamine succinate, while Bendectin contained 10 mg of doxylamine and 10 mg of vitamin B$_6$. Clinicians may choose to prescribe one Unisom and 25 mg of vitamin B$_6$ in the evening, and half a Unisom and 25 mg of vitamin B$_6$ in the morning, with good effect in many cases.

Ironically, the troubling question is whether the teratogenic effects ascribed to Bendectin are actually due to nausea and vomiting—the underlying condition for which the drug was prescribed.[23] A large study sponsored by the NIH addressed this question by reviewing data from 31,564 newborns registered in the Northern California Kaiser Permanente Birth Defects Study.[23] The investigators concluded that "there is no increase in the overall rate of major malformations after exposure to Bendectin and that the three associations found between Bendectin and individual malformations are unlikely to be causal." Fifty-eight categories of congenital malformations were reviewed in this study, and the three that were statistically associated with Bendectin exposure were microcephaly (odds ratio 5:3), congenital cataract (odds ratio 5:3), and lung malformations (odds ratio 4:6); the number of positive odds ratios reflects the number of associations that would be expected by chance. Furthermore, an independent study performed to determine whether vomiting during pregnancy in the absence of Bendectin use was associated with these three malformations found that both microcephaly and cataract were strongly associated with vomiting independent of Bendectin use. Consequently, concluded the NIH study, the underlying condition, not the drug, may be responsible for congenital malformations.

Ginger: new twist on an old remedy.   The reluctance to use drugs during early pregnancy has encouraged investigators to examine the potential value of nonmedicinal therapies. A centuries-old practice of using the fluid extract of the rhizome of ginger for symptoms of gastrointestinal distress led a Danish team to consider whether this natural product could have application in hyperemesis. Its efficacy is believed to be related to aromatic, carminative, and absorbent properties.[24] The success achieved by the Danes in 19 of 27 patients who were treated for 4 days with daily doses of 1 g of powdered rhizoma zingiberis may testify to ginger's ability to stimulate the motility of the gastrointestinal tract, thereby reducing stimuli to the chemoreceptor trigger zone. Evaluating the severity of symptoms and relief, the Danes found that 70.4% of the women gave preferential scores to the treatment period during which ginger was used compared with a placebo period.

Psychotherapeutic intervention. When carefully interviewed, patients may reveal unusual symptoms or stressors that suggest either a distinct disease process or environmental problems that need to be addressed as part of the treatment plan. A psychiatric referral is warranted when stress, anxiety, or a discrete psychopathology is suspected. Although it is uncertain what percentage of patients respond, behavioral modification, hypnosis, and brief psychotherapy have been used effectively for hyperemesis. Techniques such as stimulus deprivation, relaxation training, self-monitoring and self-control models, stimulus control, and imagery reportedly have helped in management of recurrent vomiting.[25,26]

Intriguing findings from one report suggested that patients with hyperemesis were significantly more hypnotizable than those with milder symptoms.[27] Whether hypnotherapy represents a valuable adjunct to basic psychologic support is controversial, but strong evidence of its usefulness appeared in 1980 in a study by Fuchs et al.[28] They treated 138 women with either individual or group hypnotherapy. Among the 51 patients treated individually, 69% had an excellent response, 4% a good response, and 26% a poor response. Those who underwent group hypnotherapy fared better overall: 70% showed an excellent response, 28% had a good response, and only 2% had a poor response.

References

1. Fairweather DVI. Nausea and vomiting in pregnancy. *Am J Obstet Gynecol.* 1968;102: 135–175.
2. American Council on Pharmacy and Chemistry. *JAMA.* 1956;160:208.
3. Klebanoff MA, Koslowe PA, Kaslow R, et al. Epidemiology of vomiting in early pregnancy. *Obstet Gynecol.* 1985;66:612–616.
4. Burrow SN, Ferris TF. Nausea and vomiting in pregnancy. *Medical Complications During Pregnancy.* Philadelphia, Pa: WB Saunders; 1988;304–315.
5. Brucker MC. Management of common minor discomforts in pregnancy, Part III: managing gastrointestinal problems in pregnancy. *J Nurse-Midwifery.* 1988;33:67–72.
6. Mori M, Amino N, Tamaki H, et al. Morning sickness and thyroid function in normal pregnancy. *Obstet Gynecol.* 1988;72:355–359.
7. Masson GM, Anthony F, Chau E. Serum chorionic gonadotrophin (hCG), schwangerschaftsprotein 1 (SP1), progesterone and oestradiol levels in patients with nausea and vomiting in early pregnancy. *Br J Obstet Gynaecol.* 1985;92:211.
8. Davies TF, Platzer M. HCG-induced TSH receptor activation and growth acceleration in FRTL-5 thyroid cells. *Endocrinology.* 1986;118:2149.

9. Miyai K, Tanizawa O, Yamamoto T, et al. Pituitary-thyroid function in trophoblastic disease. *J Clin Endocrinol Metab.* 1976;42:254.

10. Iatrakis GM, Sakellaropoulos GG, Kourkoubas AH, et al. Vomiting and nausea in the first 12 weeks of pregnancy. *Psychother Psychosom.* 1988;49:22–24.

11. Sahakian V, Rouse D, Sipes S, et al. Vitamin B_6 is effective therapy for nausea and vomiting of pregnancy: a randomized, double-blind placebo-controlled study. *Obstet Gynecol.* 1991;78:33–36.

12. Cleary RE, Lumeng L, Ting-Kai L. Maternal and fetal plasma levels of pyridoxine phosphate at term: adequacy of vitamin B_6 supplementation during pregnancy. *Am J Obstet Gynecol.* 1975;121:25–28.

13. O'Grady JP, Cohen LM. Emesis and hyperemesis gravidarum. In: O'Grady JP, Rosenthal M, eds. *Obstetrics: Psychological and Psychiatric Syndromes.* New York: Elsevier; 1992.

14. Fairweather DVI. Nausea and vomiting during pregnancy. *Obstet Gynecol Ann.* 1978;7:91–105.

15. Kallen B. Hyperemesis during pregnancy and delivery outcome: a registry study. *Eur J Obstet Gynecol Reprod Biol.* 1987;26:291–302.

16. Menon V, McDougall WW, Leatherdale BA. Thyrotoxic crisis following eclampsia and induction of labour. *Postgrad Med J.* 1982;58:286–287.

17. Depue RH, Bernstein L, Ross RK, et al. Hyperemesis gravidarum in relation to estradiol levels, pregnancy outcome, and other maternal factors: a seroepidemiologic study. *Am J Obstet Gynecol.* 1987;156:1137–1141.

18. Cherry SH, Merkatz I. Hyperemesis gravidarum. *Complications of Pregnancy: Medical, Surgical, Gynecologic, and Perinatal.* 4th ed. Baltimore, Md: Williams and Wilkins; 1991;220–245.

19. Gross S, Librach C, Cecutti A. Maternal weight loss associated with hyperemesis gravidarum: a predictor of fetal outcome. *Am J Obstet Gynecol.* 1989;160:906–909.

20. Chez R, Curcio FD III. Ketonuria in normal pregnancy. *Obstet Gynecol.* 1987;69:272.

21. Chin RKH, Lao TT. Low birth weight and hyperemesis gravidarum. *Eur J Obstet Gynecol Reprod Biol.* 1988;28:179–183.

22. Stellato TA, Danziger LH, Burkons D. Fetal salvage with maternal total parenteral nutrition: the pregnant mother as her own control. *J Parenter Enteral Nutr.* 1988;12:412–413.

23. Shiono PH, Klebanoff MA. Bendectin and human congenital malformations. *Teratology.* 1989;40:151–155.

24. Macy C. Psychological factors in nausea and vomiting in pregnancy: a review. *J Reprod Infant Psychol.* 1986;4:23–55.

25. Long MA, Simone S, Tucher JJ. Outpatient treatment of hyperemesis gravidarum with stimulus control and imagery procedures. *J Behav Ther Exper Psychiatry.* 1986;17:105–109.

26. Simone SS, Long MA. The behavioral treatment of hyperemesis gravidarum. *Behav Ther.* 1985;8:128–129.

27. Apfel RJ, Kelley SF, Frankel FH. The role of hypnotizability in the pathogenesis and treatment of nausea and vomiting in pregnancy. *J Psychosom Obstet Gynaecol.* 1986;5:179–186.

28. Fuchs K, Paldi, Abramovici H, et al. Treatment of hyperemesis gravidarum by hypnosis. *Int J Clin Exper Hypn.* 1980;28:313–323.

Preventing Postoperative Nausea and Vomiting

Burton S. Epstein, MD

All patients undergoing procedures that require anesthesia or sedation need to be considered potentially at risk for nausea and vomiting. These adverse events may raise questions about complications and fitness for discharge. The strikingly high incidence of nausea and vomiting in some settings—as many as 85% of patients after strabismus surgery—makes the need for more effective preventive strategies one of the overriding issues in postoperative care. Vomiting may be complicated by mild discomfort, by dehydration, or by pulmonary aspiration which potentially causes major morbidity and requires or prolongs hospitalization.

Nausea and vomiting challenge the clinical judgment of the surgical team, which should rethink its approach in initial history taking, choice of agents, techniques, routes of administration, and management in the post-anesthesia care unit (PACU). This is a multifactorial issue, related to a variety of physical, anatomic, physiologic, and pharmacologic interactions[1] (Fig 1). Its importance is underscored by retrospective studies suggesting that intractable postoperative nausea and vomiting are the leading anesthetic-related causes for unexpected hospital admission of surgical outpatients.[2]

Although a combination of new antiemetic and anesthetic agents and physical maneuvers has helped reduce the incidence of postoperative nausea and emesis, none has been entirely successful in preventing these problems and their distressing potential sequelae. More effective management strategies are needed, particularly in the ambulatory surgical theater, where both the number and the complexity of procedures performed are growing. The substantial potential cost savings of ambulatory surgery could be outweighed by unanticipated postoperative admissions for intractable nausea and vomiting. Nausea and vomiting may be the key factor in deciding whether a patient goes home.

Although postoperative nausea and vomiting remain major problems among inpatients, the importance of their management has been largely overshadowed by the dramatic growth of ambulatory procedures. Unlike inpatients, ambulatory patients are not surrounded by health care professionals

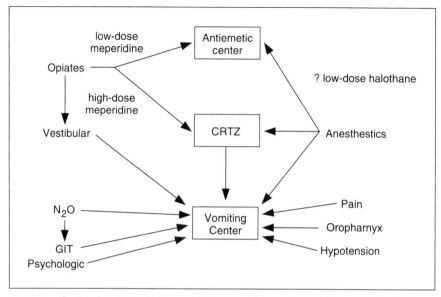

Fig 1. Anesthesia-related stimuli that can influence activity at the vomiting center, including input from the chemoreceptor trigger zone (CRTZ) and the gastrointestinal tract (GIT). (From Palazzo MGA, Strunim L. Anesthesia and emesis in etiology. *Can Anaesth Soc J.* 1984;31:78.)

and their full complement of supportive services. Nausea and vomiting could make ambulatory patients become inpatients if their suitability for discharge is not immediately and adequately addressed before, during, and after the stay in the PACU. Many management strategies used in ambulatory care are applicable to the perioperative management of inpatients. For these reasons, this discussion primarily addresses considerations for ambulatory surgery patients.

Risk Factors

Many factors predispose outpatients to develop nausea and emesis after ambulatory surgery, and some of these factors can be identified during preoperative evaluation and history taking. Patients at high risk include those predisposed to prolonged gastric emptying (e.g., patients with diabetes), those with recent food or liquid intake, patients with inadequate protective mechanisms (e.g., those with a hiatal hernia, nasogastric tube, or anesthetized upper airway), patients undergoing nausea-producing procedures such as laparoscopy, and individuals with a history of motion sickness (Table 1). The potential for emesis often can be elicited in the interview; many patients have previously experienced postoperative nausea and vomiting, and this may be their major concern about the administration of anesthesia.[3]

Table 1. Common Etiologies of Nausea and Vomiting in Outpatients

Predisposing factors	Surgical procedures
Age	Laparoscopy
Female gender	Strabismus correction
Motion sickness	Insertion of PR tubes in ears
Morbid obesity	Orchiopexy
Early pregnancy	Postoperative factors
Increased gastric volume	Hypotension
Excessive anxiety	Pain
Noncompliance	
Premedicants	
Narcotic analgesics (e.g., fentanyl)	
Anesthetic agents	
Inhaled drugs (e.g., isoflurane, N_2O)	
Intravenous drugs (e.g., etomidate)	

From White PF, Shafer A. Nausea and vomiting: causes and prophylaxis. *Sem Anesth.* 1988;6:300.

Postoperative nausea and vomiting are particularly common in children older than 2 years, and these events tend to increase in frequency with age. Both sexes are equally predisposed until puberty, when the problem becomes more common in females, a phenomenon that may be related to gonadotropin levels.

Risk assessment should also focus on the type of procedure. Patients undergoing laparoscopy, dilatation and curettage (especially for therapeutic abortion), and orchiopexy frequently develop nausea and vomiting. The incidence of vomiting following strabismus surgery is higher than that following any other outpatient surgical procedure. Generally, the longer the surgery and the period of anesthesia, the greater is the incidence of emetic symptoms.[3]

Preoperative Preparation

Physical maneuvers have been used to reduce the risk of nausea and vomiting. Such techniques include NPO regimens, preanesthetic and postanesthetic suctioning of gastric contents, and ingestion of antacid solutions.

Pressure may be applied to the cricoid cartilage during induction, and inflation of the stomach should be avoided during ventilation by mask.

Compliance with preoperative instructions is critical to the success of ambulatory surgery. Patients should be encouraged to take chronic medications on the day of surgery.[4] Recent studies tend to debunk some of the old precepts about consumption of liquids on the morning of surgery. New data suggest that prolonged liquid fasts are unnecessary in healthy patients prior to ambulatory surgery. Ingestion of coffee and pulp-free orange juice (250 mL) 2 to 3 hours before surgery apparently does not increase gastric volume. An editorial by Goresky and Waltby in a 1990 issue of the *Canadian Journal of Anaesthesia* recommends these guidelines:

(1) No solid food should be ingested on the day of surgery.

(2) Unrestricted clear liquids should be permitted until 3 hours before the scheduled time of surgery. Oral medications may be taken with 30 mL of water up to 1 hour before surgery.

(3) An H_2-blocker should be administered preoperatively to patients at increased risk of regurgitation and aspiration of gastric contents.

Anesthesia

Anesthetic Choices

The decision to use preoperative antiemetics is controversial and cannot be based solely on risk factors determined during the preoperative evaluation. The decision is partly related to whether the procedure can be performed under monitored anesthesia care (MAC) or whether a regional or a general anesthetic is required; it is also based on the degree of pain relief desired. Ultimately, the anesthesiologist must decide whether the procedure can be performed under an agent that is not likely to trigger nausea and vomiting.

Because of the reduced incidence of emesis, two studies within the last two years have indicated that propofol, which allows induction and maintenance of anesthesia with rapid recovery of consciousness, is preferred to other intravenous or inhalational methods in operations of short duration.

If a general anesthetic is required and the choice of agents includes a narcotic, the risk for nausea and vomiting is increased. In this case, preoperative administration of an antiemetic agent should be considered.

Monitored Anesthesia Care

Of all the anesthetic techniques suitable for outpatients, infiltration of the surgical site with dilute solutions of local anesthetics may be the simplest and safest technique, and the one associated with the most rapid recovery. But the injection of local anesthetics often causes severe discomfort and requires adjunctive intravenous sedative and analgesic drugs, including combinations of benzodiazepines such as midazolam and opioids such as fentanyl.[4] While the use of midazolam or propofol should not increase the risk for nausea and vomiting in MAC, analgesic requirements may dictate the administration of a narcotic, which may cause the clinician to consider the use of a preoperative antiemetic.

Regional Anesthesia

The residual analgesic action of local anesthetics may minimize the need for postoperative analgesic therapy. This presumably will decrease the need for narcotics and lower the risk for nausea and vomiting in the immediate postoperative period. However, nausea or vomiting may occur when the effects of the regional anesthetic have dissipated or the pain is treated with a narcotic.

General Anesthesia

Induction agents. The induction of general anesthesia is usually achieved with a rapid-acting intravenous drug. Those induction agents generally associated with an increased risk for postoperative nausea and vomiting include ketamine, etomidate, and the narcotics. The induction agents least likely to be associated with nausea and vomiting are propofol, thiopental, methohexital, and midazolam. With the emphasis on rapid and safe recovery for "home readiness" with a minimum of side effects, the introduction of propofol has been heralded as a significant advance.[5]

The advantages of propofol have been shown in a series of recent studies. In one study,[5] recovery was compared in two groups, one receiving propofol and nitrous oxide and the other receiving thiopentone, isoflurane, and nitrous oxide. Controlling for confounding factors, including age, sex, the nature and duration of surgery, and the use of opioid analgesics, a University of Chicago team found that the propofol-nitrous oxide regimen caused significantly fewer emetic symptoms in the PACU than thiopentone-isoflurane-nitrous oxide anesthesia. Although many procedures were laparoscopies, a procedure with a high risk for nausea and vomiting, the incidence of emesis during recovery was low in patients who received propofol and met the criteria for early discharge.[5]

Thiopental, the prototypical induction agent, produces no unique side effects when used for induction of anesthesia in outpatients.[4] In contrast, the use of methohexital is associated with hiccupping; etomidate produces pain on injection and myoclonic activity; and ketamine can produce cardiovascular stimulation during induction and excitement during emergence. Except for a higher incidence of postoperative nausea and vomiting, recovery following etomidate compares favorably with that from thiopental. While midazolam is an adequate induction agent, its onset of action is slower and recovery is prolonged compared with thiopental and methohexital.

Inhalation for induction and maintenance.   The use of a mask for inhalation induction is often associated with an increased risk for nausea and vomiting. Inhalation induction is time consuming, and many patients object to the face mask as well as the pungent smell of inhaled (volatile) agents.[4] Such risks need to be weighed against the advantages in patients without venous access and those with potential airway problems.

To maintain anesthesia, the combination of a volatile agent and nitrous oxide, 60% to 70%, is generally the technique of choice. Volatile anesthetics are frequently considered superior to intravenous anesthetics for maintenance because they are more controllable; changes in the depth of anesthesia can be made readily because of the rapid uptake or elimination of volatile agents from the lungs. In addition, the rapid elimination of anesthetic vapors usually promotes speedy recovery and an early discharge.

Propofol for maintenance of anesthesia.   Propofol is attracting interest not only for its advantages in induction but also for maintenance of anesthesia, particularly in pediatric outpatients having surgery for strabismus. A recent study from Washington University in St. Louis demonstrated the benefits of propofol in reducing the postoperative incidence of vomiting.[6] Propofol, with and without nitrous oxide and droperidol for the maintenance of anesthesia, was compared with a conventional regimen of halothane-nitrous oxide-droperidol in children undergoing elective strabismus surgery. The incidence of vomiting was reduced significantly when propofol infusion was the only agent used for maintaining anesthesia.

This does not mean that propofol has a specific antiemetic action. No data are available on the effects of propofol on the chemoreceptor trigger zone or on central dopaminergic receptors.[6] Nevertheless, an important feature of recovery from propofol anesthesia is the absence in the early recovery period of the residual "hang-over" effect often seen with use of halogenated inhalation agents. Patients receiving propofol appear to be more clear-headed and occasionally euphoric during early recovery. This could help explain their earlier ability to tolerate oral intake and to ambulate compared with patients receiving a standard inhalation anesthetic technique.

It is still uncertain whether withholding fluids and delaying ambulation affect the incidence of postoperative nausea and vomiting. Three previous reports, for example, suggest that withholding fluids and delaying ambulation may reduce the incidence of postoperative emesis. The Washington University team, however, did not find that early oral intake of fluids induced vomiting.[6]

It remains to be seen whether the incidence of emesis after maintenance of anesthesia by a total intravenous technique with propofol is decreased further by adding antiemetics, by avoiding opioids, or by inducing anesthesia with intravenous propofol.

Effect of nitrous oxide. Controversy still surrounds the role of nitrous oxide in postoperative nausea and vomiting. Apparently adding or eliminating nitrous oxide to a halothane-based regimen did not alter the incidence or severity of emesis after pediatric strabismus surgery[6] or tonsillectomy-adenoidectomy procedures.[7] In the Washington University study,[6] the addition of nitrous oxide decreased the average propofol infusion rate required to maintain satisfactory anesthesia by only 15%, but it significantly increased the incidence of vomiting. However, the investigators could not determine whether the increased emesis with propofol-nitrous oxide reflects the effect of nitrous oxide or the reduced dose of propofol.

Nevertheless, based on this study,[6] several points may be made concerning the maintenance of anesthesia in children undergoing strabismus surgery:

- Intravenous infusion of propofol after conventional induction with halothane-nitrous oxide leads to earlier recovery and a lower incidence of postoperative emesis than the standard regimen of halothane-nitrous oxide-droperidol.
- During the first 24 hours after surgery, patients receiving propofol alone have a lower incidence of emesis than those receiving propofol with nitrous oxide. However, the incidence is not less than in patients who receive droperidol with propofol and nitrous oxide.
- Patients receiving propofol alone recover and are discharged sooner than those receiving propofol-nitrous oxide-droperidol.

Another study[8] sheds additional light on the role of nitrous oxide as a potential emetic agent (Figs 2 and 3). Studying 110 inpatients undergoing elective abdominal hysterectomy, University of Chicago researchers found that nitrous oxide does not increase the incidence of nausea and vomiting.[8] Two groups of patients were compared: those who received isoflurane in either nitrous oxide and oxygen or in air and oxygen. The study confirmed a widely held clinical impression: patients were more likely to have postoperative nausea and vomiting if they had experienced nausea or vomiting after previous anesthesia.[8]

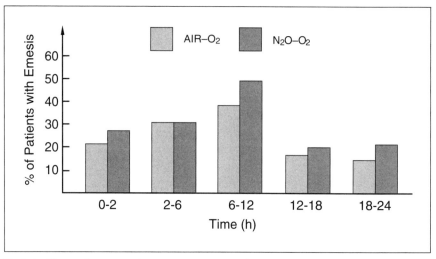

Fig 2. Incidence of postoperative emesis (nausea, retching, or vomiting) after isoflurane-air-oxygen (air-O_2) or isoflurane-nitrous oxide-oxygen (N_2O-O_2) anesthesia for abdominal hysterectomy. (From Kortilla K, et al. Nitrous oxide does not increase the incidence of nausea and vomiting after isoflurane anesthesia. *Anesth Analg.* 1987;66:761–765.)

Preoperative Prophylaxis

Whether to use prophylaxis and which therapy to employ in the treatment of nausea and vomiting remain controversial issues.[9] Although anesthesiologists tend to rely less and less on preoperative antiemetic agents, certain risk factors may suggest that they are needed. Patient-related factors, particularly predisposition, are often decisive. If a patient reports a history of intractable vomiting, possibly requiring hospital admission, every time an anesthetic is administered, preoperative use of antiemetic agents should be strongly considered. Both a history of motion sickness and the type of procedure may determine whether prophylaxis is called for. Laparoscopic procedures and strabismus surgery, for example, notoriously increase the risk. These factors—in addition to the induction agent and the possible use of narcotics for induction, maintenance, or postoperative analgesia—are important considerations in determining the need for prophylaxis.

If prophylaxis is required, what are the appropriate choices? To what extent are they effective? Current approaches include the following:

- Preoperative use of droperidol, shown to reduce the incidence of vomiting prior to discharge by as much as 50%.[10]
- Preoperative administration of metoclopramide.
- Placement of a transdermal scopolamine patch several hours before surgery.

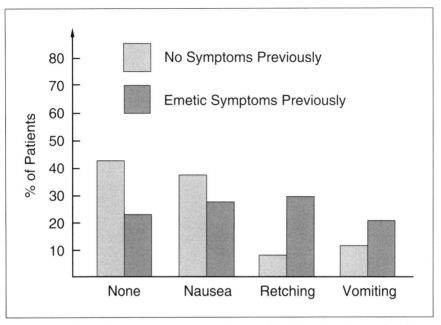

Fig 3. The incidence of postoperative nausea, retching, and vomiting in patients undergoing abdominal hysterectomy under general anesthesia. Some patients had nausea or vomiting after previous anesthetics (n = 44), and others had no nausea or vomiting after previous anesthetics (n = 53). (From Kortilla K, et al. Nitrous oxide does not increase the incidence of nausea and vomiting after isoflurane anesthesia. *Anesth Analg.* 1987;66:761–765.)

- Use of ephedrine in patients undergoing general anesthesia for outpatient laparoscopy, particularly as prophylaxis for patients prone to motion sickness or for those in whom dizziness, nausea, and/or vomiting occur postoperatively upon ambulation.

Droperidol. Droperidol is believed to reduce the incidence of postoperative emesis more than any other treatment. Studies of strabismus surgery have demonstrated the efficacy of intravenous droperidol, 75 mcg/kg to unpremedicated children at the time of induction and before manipulation of the extraocular muscles.[11]

One question surrounding the use of droperidol is whether its sedative effects might unreasonably prolong discharge time. University of Pennsylvania investigators[10] advanced the theory that preoperative use of droperidol would reduce the incidence of emesis and not prolong discharge time if it were administered early, as a component of oral premedication. The rationale underlying the selection of droperidol was simple: to retain the desirable properties of the premedication and to decrease the incidence of postoperative emesis without introducing any adverse effects. In this study,

65 patients were randomized to receive one of three premedication regimens: (1) standard oral premedication, consisting of meperidine, diazepam, and atropine; (2) a 50 μg/kg dose of droperidol instead of diazepam; and (3) a 75 μg/kg dose of droperidol instead of diazepam. Both doses of droperidol produced sedative effects comparable to a 0.15 mg/kg dose of diazepam. As expected, the sedative effect did not differ among the three study groups, but the droperidol-treated groups had a significantly lower incidence of vomiting prior to hospital discharge (33% in the low-dose group and 36% in the high-dose group).[10]

Droperidol appeared to be most effective during the early postoperative period, when the incidence of vomiting was 0% and 14% in the high- and low-dose groups, respectively, compared with a 55% incidence in children receiving the standard oral premedication. In the later postoperative period, fewer differences could be found among the treatment groups. By the time children reached the day-surgery unit, the incidence of vomiting was still lower in the droperidol groups compared with the standard premedication group, but the difference was not statistically significant. From discharge to the morning after the procedure, even fewer differences were found among the three groups. One reason may be that the control group received other antiemetics, while patients given droperidol did not.[10]

The advantages of administering droperidol before strabismus surgery were confirmed by Canadian investigators who studied use of the agent in 100 children randomly assigned to one of three treatment groups: intravenous droperidol, rectal acetaminophen, or intramuscular codeine.[11] It is apparent from this study and others that droperidol is most effective in strabismus surgery if administered before manipulation of the eye, which is the stimulus to vomit. To reduce the risk of vomiting after strabismus repair to a clinically acceptable level, intravenous droperidol should be given at induction of anesthesia (about 10 minutes before manipulation of the eye).

Investigators still disagree, however, on the optimal dose of droperidol for prophylaxis. A recent study[12] evaluating a range of doses found an inverse relationship between the size of the dose and occurrence of nausea and vomiting. But larger doses of the drug were also associated with residual sedative effects, which can delay the emergence from general anesthesia.[12] The recommendation of a 0.6 mg intravenous dose of droperidol for the adult represents a compromise between reduction in the incidence of emesis and postoperative sedation.[13]

Metoclopramide. The profound and prolonged sedation often associated with large doses of droperidol, which may delay discharge and require an unscheduled hospital admission, has encouraged study of alternatives. Metoclopramide is an antiemetic drug with a relatively short duration of action, and its nonsedating qualities could offer distinct advantages in the outpatient surgery setting. The drug increases lower esophageal sphincter pressure and the rate of gastric emptying.

A study conducted at the Children's Hospital, University of California, San Diego, assessed the prophylactic effect of metoclopramide when administered preoperatively to patients undergoing strabismus surgery and directly compared the activity of metoclopramide and droperidol in this particularly vulnerable ambulatory population.[14] The results, based on the recovery of 79 patients, indicated that a 0.25 mg/kg dose of metoclopramide was as effective as droperidol in preventing postoperative vomiting. Hospital stays were not prolonged with the use of either drug.[14]

Transdermal scopolamine. The safety and efficacy of transdermal scopolamine has aroused growing interest in view of recent studies suggesting it may have an expanded role as an antiemetic in the preoperative or postoperative setting. Scopolamine blocks cholinergic stimulation of the vomiting center from both the gastrointestinal tract and the vestibular center. When the drug is delivered intramuscularly or intravenously, it produces relatively high plasma concentrations which frequently result in undesirable side effects, such as excessive sedation, agitation, and hallucinations. Another problem encountered with the parenteral form of the drug is its short elimination half-life, approximately 1 hour.

The development of a transdermal delivery system that continuously releases scopolamine for up to 3 days means that low steady-state plasma concentrations are available. Such low concentrations, providing more consistent antiemetic action with fewer side effects, have prompted investigators to evaluate use of transdermal scopolamine in patients undergoing laparoscopy. A recent study enrolling 191 women at the University of Utah suggests the potential value of transdermal scopolamine for this procedure.[15] This study confirmed several other reports, including one documenting its advantages in patients undergoing major gynecologic surgery. However, the transdermal scopolamine system has been reported to produce bizarre behavior when administered to children prior to strabismus surgery.[16]

In the Utah study,[15] anesthesia was induced with fentanyl, thiopental, and succinylcholine and maintained with isoflurane and nitrous oxide in oxygen. Scopolamine-treated patients had less nausea, retching, and vomiting than placebo-treated patients. Severe nausea and vomiting were reported in 62% of the placebo group but in only 37% of patients with the transdermal system. Repeated episodes of retching and vomiting were also less frequent in the scopolamine group (23% vs. 41%). Patients on scopolamine tended to be discharged earlier. Although side effects were more common with the scopolamine patch, they were not considered troublesome.

It may be that eliminating fentanyl and nitrous oxide helped reduce the incidence of postoperative nausea and vomiting. Perhaps other antiemetic agents, such as droperidol, are as effective as the scopolamine patch. However, other parenterally administered agents probably will not provide as long-lasting relief as transdermal scopolamine.[15]

Although scattered reports suggest that the patch may be associated with hallucinations or extreme agitation in some patients, especially children, acceptance by adult patients is generally high. The patch should be applied at least several hours before surgery to maximize its efficacy. It appears to be most beneficial in patients at high risk for nausea and vomiting, including those with a history of significant postoperative nausea and vomiting and patients undergoing procedures known to produce a high incidence of this problem.[15]

Ephedrine.   Although not as well established within the spectrum of therapy as other antiemetic agents, ephedrine is generating interest based on new evidence that bolsters anecdotal reports of its efficacy in the prevention of nausea and vomiting. A sympathomimetic drug, ephedrine was used initially because it minimized motion sickness when given in combination with scopolamine, and it reduced the latter's sedative effects.[17] After a study indicated that ephedrine has antiemetic effects when used alone, investigators more closely examined its pharmacokinetic action.

The antiemetic effects of sympathomimetic drugs are indirectly supported by appearance of symptoms that mimic motion sickness when subjects are given phenoxybenzamine, a sympatholytic drug. A high degree of vagal tone in the perioperative period may contribute to nausea and vomiting, and ephedrine may minimize these symptoms by increasing sympathetic tone.[17] Ephedrine also may act in other ways to reduce the incidence of nausea and vomiting. The hypotension that accompanies spinal or epidural anesthesia is often heralded by nausea and vomiting, due to a reduction in medullary blood flow to the chemoreceptor trigger zone. Ephedrine is commonly used to increase mean arterial pressure and, presumably, medullary blood flow as well, thus minimizing these symptoms.[17]

Researchers speculate that ephedrine may be able to minimize nausea and vomiting associated with postural hypotension after outpatient surgery. Postural hypotension may occur after general anesthesia, especially with ambulation, due to depletion of intravascular volume or to residual vasodilation from anesthetics.

Adjunctive Anesthesia

Outpatient surgical procedures of short duration (1 hour or less) were frequently performed under a light-plane anesthetic, such as a combination of nitrous oxide in oxygen and thiopental.[18] Patients anesthetized with these agents are readily stimulated by the pain of surgical incisions or visceral manipulation.

We studied the advantages and disadvantages of adding fentanyl to thiopental combined with nitrous oxide in oxygen to determine whether this potent, short-acting narcotic analgesic provided a smoother course of anesthesia and reduced the requirements for thiopental without increasing recovery time. The surgical procedures were dilatation and curettage and voluntary interruption of pregnancy. A high frequency of nausea and vomiting was not expected with the use of fentanyl. Even though the incidence of nausea and vomiting was high in the immediate postoperative period, there was no statistically significant difference between the fentanyl and placebo-treated groups. The need for antiemetic medication also did not differ between groups.

Discharge Criteria and Postoperative Prophylaxis
Although a variety of tests have been devised to assess central nervous system recovery and "home readiness" following general anesthesia, there are no standardized discharge criteria.[4] The patient must be awake and oriented to person, place, and time, with stable vital signs for at least 30 to 60 minutes. He or she must be able to ambulate without assistance, and pain should be adequately controlled with oral analgesics. Toleration of oral fluids prior to discharge is less frequently considered a requirement for discharge. Indeed, forcing fluids early in the postoperative period may increase the incidence of nausea and vomiting.

Postoperative complications and side effects that commonly delay discharge and result in unexpected admissions include excessive bleeding or pain, prolonged emergence, dizziness, and intractable vomiting.[4] Among the more important suggested guidelines regarding vomiting are the following:

- Ambulatory patients who have persistent nausea and vomiting while supine but who have not taken any oral fluids and who are not in pain should receive an antiemetic.
- Patients in pain should be given a narcotic analgesic, recognizing the increased risk of nausea and vomiting, unless a nonnarcotic analgesic will suffice.
- If patients vomit only with administration of oral fluids, they should be discontinued; intravenous fluids should be relied upon for hydration.
- Patients who vomit only when they change positions may benefit from ephedrine; it is useful in helping patients make the transition between the supine and upright positions.
- Droperidol should be used when indicated, in the smallest dose

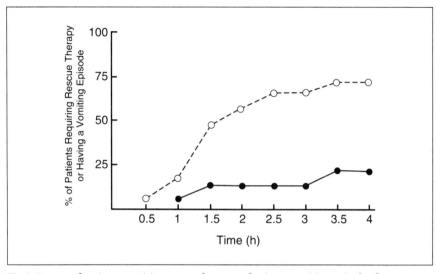

Fig 4. Percent of patients requiring rescue therapy or having a vomiting episode after administration; placebo (open circles); ondansetron (solid circles). (From Larijani GE, et al. Treatment of postoperative nausea and vomiting with ondansetron: a randomized double-blind comparison with placebo. *Anesth Analg.* 1991;73:246–249.)

possible, 10 µg/kg to 20 µg/kg. If it needs to be readministered, a higher dose (50 µg/kg to 75 µg/kg) should be reserved for intractable cases.

- Scopolamine should be used preoperatively rather than postoperatively. However, the frequency of bizzare central nervous system reactions speaks against its use in children. Metoclopramide (0.15 mg/kg to 0.25 mg/kg) may be a better choice, especially in the PACU.

The Potential Role of Ondansetron

Although primarily studied for its use in chemotherapy-induced emesis, ondansetron is generating interest for preventing perioperative nausea and emesis. Its success in the treatment of cytotoxic chemotherapy-induced emesis has led several groups to investigate its role in surgical patients (Fig 4). Unlike most commonly used antiemetic medications, ondansetron is devoid of activity at dopaminergic, histaminergic, adrenergic, and cholinergic receptors. Consequently, it is unlikely to cause side effects such as hypotension, sedation, restlessness, dysphoria, and the extrapyramidal symptoms associated with other antiemetic agents.

The lack of side effects was apparent in a recent study at Washington University, St. Louis, in which ondansetron (8 mg administered intravenously) was significantly more effective than placebo in treating postoperative nausea and vomiting in outpatients undergoing laparoscopic procedures.[2] Of the 155 patients studied, 51% of those treated with ondansetron experienced subsequent episodes of vomiting in the PACU, compared with 92% of the control group given saline. Only 43% of ondansetron-treated patients needed a "rescue" antiemetic, compared with 86% of those treated with placebo. The rescue combination consisted of metoclopramide and hydroxyzine. Ondansetron probably is as effective as the combination of metoclopramide and hydroxyzine, according to the Washington University team.

Because the use of ondansetron is still investigational and controversial in the surgical setting, further studies are needed to determine the optimal dose for both treatment and prevention of emetic sequelae.[2] In contrast to the nausea associated with specific cytotoxic chemotherapeutic agents that trigger serotonin release, perioperative nausea and emesis may be a multifactorial issue related to a variety of physical, anatomic, physiologic, and pharmacologic interactions. Nevertheless, if it can be shown that ondansetron, either alone or in combination with other agents with different mechanisms of action, can improve the effectiveness of antiemetic management, physicians will have a potent option that dramatically expands the spectrum of therapy. Absence of vomiting at the time of discharge is no assurance that vomiting will not occur after discharge.

Droperidol vs. Metoclopramide

Anesthesiologists may be reluctant to use an antiemetic such as droperidol because of prolonged drowsiness. However, somnolence may be less important than vomiting in delaying discharge.[19] Although 4 to 6 hours from surgery to discharge might be considered prolonged recovery in children after myringotomy or herniotomy, this amount of time is common after surgical procedures such as orchiopexy and strabismus correction. Reduction in the frequency and severity of vomiting within an acceptable period for same-day discharge is important.

Higher doses of droperidol may be called for in certain situations. For example, the incidence of vomiting in children undergoing strabismus surgery decreased from 85% in a placebo group to 43% in a group receiving droperidol 75 μg/kg.[19] This dose also reduced the severity of vomiting; no patient who received droperidol prophylactically required its therapeutic use.[19]

Mounting evidence suggests that metoclopramide may be preferable to droperidol as a postoperative antiemetic because of its relatively short duration of action and lack of sedation.[20] Metoclopramide probably reduces postoperative nausea and vomiting through several mechanisms. Like droperidol, it is a dopamine antagonist, which means its antiemetic effects are probably mediated, at least in part, by blockade of dopamine receptors in the chemoreceptor trigger zone. In addition, metoclopramide increases lower esophageal sphincter tone and is probably active through acetylcholine receptors. Yet the most important peripheral antiemetic effect of metoclopramide may be its ability to increase gastric motor activity. This effect probably prevents gastric relaxation, which must precede vomiting. Recent evidence suggests that metoclopramide, 0.15 mg/kg administered at the completion of strabismus surgery, is the most effective dose.

The Challenge of Finding New and More Effective Strategies

Postoperative care has significantly reduced the risks of nausea and vomiting following ambulatory surgery, but in many situations recovery times are still too long and the incidence of side effects remains too high.[4] The therapy of last resort, hospitalization, is ultimately unsatisfactory for the patient, the anesthesiologist, and the surgeon. As the number of operations performed in the outpatient setting grows and as more older and sicker patients present for more complex procedures, the need for more sophisticated management strategies and approaches will also grow. However, advances in anesthetic techniques that promote earlier recovery—such as the wider use of propofol—and new, potentially important developments in antiemetic prophylaxis (including ondansetron) may signify dramatic changes that will shorten recovery times and prevent complications that delay discharge. We need these and other innovative and effective approaches to meet the challenge of developing techniques that further reduce the rate of unexpected hospital admissions.

References

1. Kapur PA. Editorial: the big "little problem." *Anesth Analg.* 1991;73:243–245.
2. Bodner M, White P. Antiemetic efficacy of ondansetron after outpatient laparoscopy. *Anesth Analg.* 1991;73:250–254.
3. Kallar SK, Jones GW. Postoperative complications. In: White PF, ed. *Outpatient Anesthesia.* New York: Churchill Livingstone; 1990:397–415.
4. White PF. Patient selection and anesthetic techniques for the ambulatory patients. Annual Refresher Course Lectures. American Society of Anesthesiolgists; 1991;512:1–7.
5. Kortilla K, Ostman P, Faure E, et al. Randomized comparison of recovery after propofol-nitrous oxide versus thiopentone-isoflurane-nitrous oxide anaesthesia in patients undergoing ambulatory surgery. *Acta Anaesthesiol Scand.* 1990;34:400–403.
6. Watcha MF, Simeon RM, White PF, et al. Effect of propofol on the incidence of postoperative vomiting after strabismus surgery in pediatric outpatients. *Anesthesiology.* 1991;75:204–209.

7. Pandit U, Pryn S, Randel G, et al. Nitrous oxide does not increase postoperative nausea/vomiting in pediatric outpatients undergoing tonsillectomy-adenoidectomy. *Anesthesiology.* 1990;67:A1245.

8. Kortilla K, Hovorka J, Erkola O. Nitrous oxide does not increase the incidence of nausea and vomiting after isoflurane anesthesia. *Anesth Analg.* 1987;66:761–765.

9. Epstein B. Controversial aspects of ambulatory surgery: recovery and discharge. *Anesth Rev.* 1990;17:39–44.

10. Nicolson SC, Kaya KM, Betts EK. The effect of preoperative oral droperidol on the incidence of postoperative emesis after paediatric strabismus surgery. *Can J Anaesth.* 1988;35:364–367.

11. Lerman J, Eustis S, Smith DR. Effect of droperidol pretreatment on postanesthetic vomiting in children undergoing strabismus surgery. *Anesthesiology.* 1986;65:322–325.

12. Poler SM, White PF, Margrabe D, et al. Nausea and vomiting in outpatients—use of droperidol prophylaxis. *Anesthesiology.* 1989;71:A134.

13. Wetchler BV, Collins IS, Jacob L. Antiemetic effects of droperidol on the ambulatory surgery patient. *Anesth Rev.* 1982;9:23.

14. Lin DM, Furst, SR, Rodarte A. A double-blinded comparison of metoclopramide and droperidol for prevention of emesis following strabismus surgery. *Anesthesiology.* 1992;76:357–361.

15. Bailey PL, Streisand JB, Pace NL. Transdermal scopolamine reduces nausea and vomiting after outpatient laparoscopy. *Anesthesiology.* 1990;72:977–980.

16. Gibbons PA, Nicolson SC, Betts EK, et al. Scopolamine does not prevent post-operative emesis after pediatric eye surgery. *Anesthesiology.* 1984;61:A435.

17. Rothenberg DM, Parnass SM, Litwack K, et al. Efficacy of ephedrine in the prevention of postoperative nausea and vomiting. *Anesth Analg.* 1991;72:58–61.

18. Epstein BS, Levy M-L, Thein MH, et al. Evaluation of fentanyl as an adjunct to thiopental-nitrous oxide-oxygen anesthesia for short surgical procedures. *Anesth Rev.* 1975:24–29.

19. Abramowitz MD, Oh TH, Epstein BS, et al. The antiemetic effect of droperidol following outpatient strabismus surgery in children. *Anesthesiology.* 1983;59:579–583.

20. Broadman LM, Ceruzzi W, Patane PS, et al. Metoclopramide reduces the incidence of vomiting following strabismus surgery in children. *Anesthesiology.* 1990;72:245–248.

Radiation-Induced Nausea and Vomiting

T. J. Priestman, MD

Despite their major role in patient compliance, radiation-induced nausea and vomiting have undergone limited scientific and clinical research. In contrast to the vast literature on chemotherapy-induced emesis, the data base on radiation-induced emesis is relatively small. Until recently, physiologic disturbances after total-body irradiation had been studied only in victims of nuclear war, weapon-testing accidents, or industrial misadventures.[1] Because these circumstances involve uncontrolled exposure, the precise effects of total dosage, dose rate, and radiation quality were difficult to determine. Recent studies, however, have begun to elucidate the relationship between radiation and nausea and vomiting and are delineating factors that help to predict the likelihood that such sickness will develop during treatment.

Although most patients undergoing radiotherapy as part of treatment for cancer do not develop nausea and vomiting, a substantial minority are affected. Particularly affected are patients having high-dose, large-volume irradiation, such as total-body irradiation prior to bone marrow transplantation (Figs 1 and 2). In this subset of patients, nausea and vomiting are significant problems, requiring a range of prophylactic strategies. Generally, the degree of emesis associated with radiotherapy is less severe than emesis associated with cisplatin-based chemotherapy, but the sickness may be of much longer duration, depending on the course of radiotherapy.

A comprehensive literature search on postirradiation nausea and vomiting suggests that three interrelated factors most strongly influence whether a patient will develop these problems:

- The volume of tissue irradiated is an important predictor of sickness. Total-body irradiation is associated with severe nausea and vomiting in virtually every patient.
- When the radiation field includes the upper part of the gut, emesis is common. When the treatment is restricted to other sites, nausea and vomiting may still occur, but less predictably.

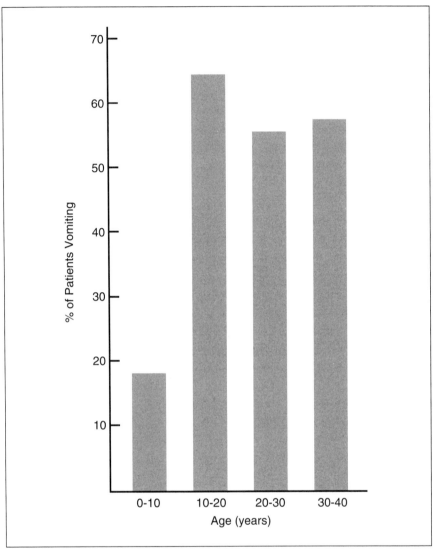

Fig 1. Percent of patients vomiting when treated with whole-body irradiation, by age. (From Westbrook C, et al. Vomiting associated with whole body irradiation. *Clin Radiol.* 1987;38:263–266.)

- The dose of irradiation is also a powerful predictor of the likelihood of emesis. The risk of sickness increases steadily as the dose in a single treatment exceeds 2 Gy.

Two other factors—age and anxiety—have been identified as potentially important variables in predicting sickness. Children are reportedly less susceptible to radiation-induced emesis than adults. The role of anxiety needs more study to elucidate its impact on emesis.

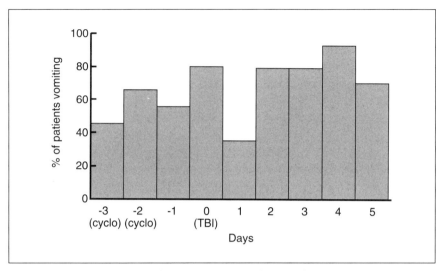

Fig 2. Vomiting in association with bone marrow transplantation for patients with leukemia receiving total-body irradiation (TBI) with a single-source cobalt unit. (From Westbrook C, et al. Vomiting associated with whole body irradiation. *Clin Radiol.* 1987;38:263–266.)

The term "prodromal effects" refers to the symptoms of emesis, nausea, and malaise that appear on the day of radiation therapy, typically presenting 2 hours after treatment.[2] Vomiting and diarrhea may occur 1 to 3 days after treatment in patients exposed to lethal doses of radiation, due to the degenerative effects of such exposure. The term "radiation sickness" covers all sequelae, including signs and symptoms that may persist for several weeks.[2]

Mechanisms.   The precise mechanisms of radiation-induced emesis are unclear, but investigators postulate that it may be attributable either to the direct effect of radiation damage to the gut or to the release of chemicals from the gut that influence the vomiting center. The concepts derived from animal models could help explain the pathophysiology of emesis following radiotherapy. It is widely believed that nausea and vomiting are controlled by the area postrema, a circumventricular organ near the caudal floor of the fourth cerebral ventricle. Highly vascular and outside the blood-brain barrier, the area postrema contains the chemoreceptor trigger zone, which mediates the stimuli provided by emetic compounds borne in blood or cerebrospinal fluid.[2] These stimuli may be relayed to a vomiting center nearby in the reticular formation of the medulla.[2] The model also includes visceral afferents, both vagal and splanchnic, that project to the vomiting center.

A humoral substance acting at the area postrema may be directly implicated in the development of radiation-induced conditioned taste aversion in rats, an analogue model of nausea in this species that lacks a vomiting response.[3] Intravenous injections of certain peptides induce vomiting in dogs, and the area postrema is necessary for this response.[4] Wu et al[5] demonstrated that some of the same peptides induce vomiting when placed in the cerebrospinal fluid bathing the area postrema. When these findings are considered with other data, the role of the area postrema in various humorally mediated events looks more convincing. The "humoral hypothesis" is further supported by animal studies indicating that ablation of the area postrema inhibits radiation-induced vomiting.[6]

Nevertheless, another school of thought suggesting that visceral afferents are more important has emerged. The impetus for this view is older investigations demonstrating that supradiaphragmatic vagotomy in the monkey significantly reduces radiation-induced vomiting.[7] Ablation of the area postrema enhanced this effect. In more recent studies, discrete lesions were made in the area postrema, abolishing radiation-induced vomiting in the dog.[8] Although these findings are provocative and favor the role of visceral afferents, the issue is still unsettled.

According to Harding,[2] the area postrema is the most sensitive site for reception of emetic stimuli. However, visceral receptors play a secondary role, apparent in studies involving dogs in which the area postrema was ablated.[9] Previous work suggested that such ablation would completely inhibit emesis following a radiation dose of 6 Gy to 8 Gy. However, these animals, whose visceral emetic reflex remained intact after area postrema ablation, vomited when they were exposed to a dose of 15 Gy to 20 Gy.[9] Therefore, the neuronal (visceral) pathway appears to exist in parallel with the area postrema or humoral mechanism, but the latter is more sensitive (Fig 3).[2] Further proof of their different sensitivity is provided by the work of Carpenter et al,[10] who found that vagotomy did not affect emesis induced by abdominal radiation of 8 Gy.

Total-Body Irradiation

Total-body irradiation may be delivered in multiple fractions or as a single exposure, whereas hemibody irradiation is usually given as a single treatment.[1] A study in 305 patients undergoing total-body irradiation indicated the patterns of vomiting and the role of different fraction sizes in provoking emesis[1] (Fig 4). The study group had acute lymphatic or myeloid leukemia, and the progress would have been poor if conventional chemotherapy had been used alone. The incidence of vomiting peaked 4 days after total-body irradiation, and vomiting was often associated with diarrhea. Vomiting usually began after administration of a dose of 2 Gy to 3 Gy; in some cases, it persisted for up to 12 hours. Patients vomited infrequently, however,

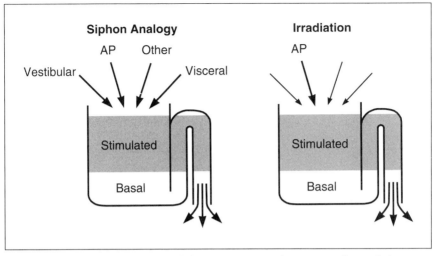

Fig 3. Siphon analogy for vomiting. *Left,* four main sources of emetic stimuli: vestibular; area postrema (AP) stimulation provided by substances borne in blood and cerebrospinal fluid and by interneurons; other: supramedullary stimuli; visceral: carried by vagal and splanchnic afferents. These may separately or in combination provide stimuli, which upon reaching a threshold lead to an emetic response. *Right,* particular emetic stimuli, such as irradiation, may act predominantly through one of the four main input sources; however, other sources may also contribute. (From Harding RK. Prodromal effects of radiation: pathways, models, and protection by antiemetics. *Pharm Ther.* 1988;39:335–345.)

with fractionated radiation of less than 2 Gy. Once the threshold for emesis had been reached, the cumulative dose was not a decisive factor. For example, no vomiting was observed in 10 young children treated with fractionated whole-body irradiation (6 fractions of 2 Gy at a higher dose rate over 3 days). Vomiting was more likely to interrupt treatment when patients were treated with single-source cobalt 60 and with cyclophospha-mide rather than with melphalan. Vomiting may have been reduced with melphalan because it was given immediately before irradiation, and its emetic effect may have been delayed[1]; cyclophosphamide was administered a day before patients underwent radiotherapy. When sedation was used in restless patients, it was more effective in those treated with the dual than with the single source cobalt 60 unit, probably because they experienced less discomfort.

Use of the dual-head cobalt 60 unit could be a significant variable in view of the reduced incidence of vomiting associated with it. Compared with the single-source cobalt 60 unit, the dual head may provide greater comfort, thereby reducing psychological strain and limiting patient movement.

Insufficient data prevented this study from analyzing the role of susceptibility to motion sickness. However, there was a strong clinical

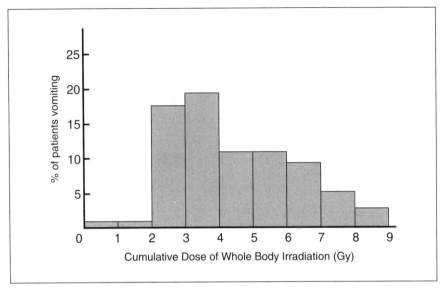

Fig 4. Incidence of vomiting in 107 patients treated with single-source cobalt unit. (From Westbrook C, et al. Vomiting associated with whole body irradiation. *Clin Radiol.* 1987;38:263–266.)

impression that patients were more prone to vomit when exposed to other precipitating factors, including anxiety. This implies that the vestibular apparatus and higher centers play major roles in the induction of vomiting by whole-body irradiation.

The reduced incidence of vomiting in children younger than 10 years (Fig 1) is probably related to psychological factors. Young children are relatively unaware of the significance of their treatment and its ramifications. So long as the treatment is not painful and they are reassured about their attendants and surroundings, they are not apt to experience much anxiety. Older children are more prone to anxiety because they understand the life-threatening nature of their disease but may be ill-equipped to cope with it compared with adults.[1]

Further evidence that emesis can be expected in virtually every patient undergoing total-body irradiation, even when small-dose fractions are used, came from another recent study. The 29 patients underwent radiotherapy as the initial phase of conditioning for bone marrow transplantation. The total radiation dose was 1320 cGy, given as 11 fractions of 120 cGy over 4 days at a rate of 22 cGy/min. Despite the use of antiemetic regimens in 23 of the 29 patients, the mean number of emetic episodes was 3.0, 1.8, 1.3, and 1.1 on days 1, 2, 3, and 4 of treatment. Emesis occurred uniformly despite small dose fractions and was not related to a cumulative dose.

Site

It has long been recognized that patients undergoing radiotherapy to the upper abdomen are at greatest risk for emesis. The degree of risk was demonstrated by one report involving patients undergoing hemibody irradiation.[12] After receiving single doses of 8 Gy without prophylactic antiemetics, 91% of the patients having upper body irradiation and 33% receiving lower body treatment had significant emesis.

The emesis may be related to the release of substances such as methionine, catecholamines, prostaglandins, dopamine, and enkephalin, which provoke vomiting by stimulating the chemoreceptor trigger zone. Nevertheless, a significant minority of patients experience emesis with irradiation of sites where such mechanisms cannot be implicated.

Dosage

Patients undergoing curative radiotherapy generally receive treatment 5 days a week for 3 to 8 weeks. Most patients undergo daily treatment with 1.8 Gy to 3 Gy, and the risk of emesis steadily increases when the dose reaches at least 2 Gy. Emesis is very likely if more than 8 Gy is administered. Patients receiving palliative radiation frequently have a single exposure of 8 Gy to 15 Gy.

Antiemetic Therapy

Prophylactic antiemetic therapy is not indicated for most patients undergoing radiotherapy. The decision to administer such treatment is largely dictated by the interrelationships among the three leading risk factors—volume of tissue irradiated, site, and dose. For example, patients undergoing a single treatment with 8 Gy or more to the upper abdomen would be prime candidates for consideration of prophylactic antiemetic therapy.

Until recently, oral metoclopramide was considered first-line therapy in this situation. Patients typically receive 10 mg three times a day starting an hour or two before irradiation. Because similar mechanisms are thought to be involved in the pathogenesis of radiation-induced and chemotherapy-induced nausea and vomiting,[13] investigators have postulated that some of the same antiemetic agents effective in patients undergoing chemotherapy could have application for patients undergoing radiotherapy.

Nabilone, for example, has been shown to be an effective drug in the management of chemotherapy-induced emesis and has demonstrated superiority over prochlorperazine.[14] A pilot study of nabilone—in which a 2 mg daily dose was found effective in patients refractory to metoclopramide—prompted us to continue comparing these agents as first-line drugs for nausea and vomiting caused by radiotherapy.[15]

In this randomized, double-blind, crossover study,[15] 20 patients received nabilone and 19 received metoclopramide. Patients qualified for the study if they had at least five treatments remaining in their planned course of irradiation. When patients were asked to rate the efficacy of the antiemetic treatment as good, adequate, or poor, no significant differences were found between the two agents. Most patients reported that both drugs controlled nausea and vomiting but did not completely eradicate the symptoms. Nabilone caused significantly greater toxicity, although another report suggests that adverse effects may be overcome if the drug is combined with prochlorperazine.[16] Overall, metoclopramide appears to be the better choice as first-line therapy.

Although a number of studies have explored the use of cannabinoids such as nabilone to reduce the nausea and vomiting caused by cytotoxic drugs, few studies have addressed whether this class of agents might benefit patients undergoing radiotherapy. A pilot study[17] comparing the cannabis derivative levonantradol and chlorpromazine did not find significant differences between these treatments in 43 patients who received palliative, single-fraction radiotherapy to sites near the upper abdomen. Approximately one half of all patients vomited, regardless of treatment. It remains to be seen whether higher doses of levonantradol or other cannabinoids might be more effective. After a short-lived popularity in the 1980s for the treatment of radiation-induced emesis, cannabinoids do not appear to have fulfilled the early promise predicted for them, failing largely because of toxicity rather than because of lack of efficacy.

Prochlorperazine, however, may be an alternative to metoclopramide, according to results in a study involving outpatients who received radiotherapy to the thorax or abdomen.[18] Of the 89 patients studied, 28 received metoclopramide (100 mg every 4 hours), 30 received prochlorperazine (10 mg every 4 hours), and 31 received placebo. No statistically significant differences were found among the treatment groups after the first two doses, based on a diary of symptoms kept by the patients and the global impression of the investigators. Although an argument can be made for lack of efficacy of both antiemetics, the numbers in each arm of the study were too small to draw negative conclusions. A clear difference in toxicity was noted between treatments, with 21 adverse experiences with metoclopramide and 6 adverse experiences with prochlorperazine. But it must be remembered that the dose of metoclopramide was particularly high for a radiotherapy study. This is the only published report on the use of prochlorperazine in the control of radiation-induced emesis. Despite the paucity of trial data the drug remains a popular agent in clinical practice.

5-HT$_3$ Receptor Antagonists

The prevention of vomiting in only half of patients undergoing treatment with conventional antiemetics following total-body irradiation or radiotherapy of the upper abdomen highlights the need for more effective strategies. One of the exciting avenues of therapeutic research is the development of a new class of agents, the 5-hydroxytryptamine$_3$ (5-HT$_3$) receptor antagonists.

The rationale for use of this class of drugs is based on work showing that radiation damage to the gastrointestinal mucosa releases 5-HT$_3$.[19] The 5-HT$_3$ then initiates the vomiting reflex by activating 5-HT$_3$ receptors located centrally in the area postrema on peripheral afferent nerves which project into the area postrema.[20] In contrast to antiemetics such as metoclopramide, the agents in this class are devoid of dopamine receptor antagonism. Paralleling antiemetic research on the use of 5-HT$_3$ receptor antagonists such as ondansetron in chemotherapy-induced emesis, investigators have demonstrated that such agents are effective in preventing sickness following radiotherapy.

At many centers, metoclopramide has been the most widely used agent for control of radiation-induced nausea and vomiting. Clinicians are now reconsidering its role as a first-line agent in view of new data comparing its efficacy with that of ondansetron.

A recent report[21] compared these two agents in prevention of sickness after single-exposure radiation treatments of 8 Gy to 10 Gy to the upper abdomen.[21] One day after irradiation, ondansetron prevented vomiting or retching in all but 1 of 38 patients, whereas metoclopramide completely controlled symptoms in only 46% of 44 patients ($P<0.001$). Ondansetron was also superior in preventing nausea. On day 1, 95% of patients given ondansetron graded their nausea as absent or mild and none experienced severe nausea; in comparison, 20% of patients on metoclopramide experiencing severe nausea. After the first day, ondansetron achieved complete controlled or major control (<2 episodes) of vomiting and retching in 92% to 100% of patients. The antiemetic efficacy was maintained up to the fifth and last study day. Metoclopramide achieved equivalent control in 70% of patients on the first day and 95% on day 5. The improved efficacy with time probably reflects the waning of the emetic stimulus after irradiation. Both agents were well tolerated, with no major side effects or problems with compliance. A final report,[22] including an additional 15 evaluable patients, confirmed the results of the earlier series.[21] Complete control of emesis in the first 20 hours after radiotherapy was achieved in 92% of ondansetron patients compared with 46% of the metoclopramide group ($P<0.001$). Nausea was absent or mild in 88% of patients given on-dansetron and in 60% of those on metoclopramide ($P=0.001$).[22]

Encouraged by these results, we conducted a further prospective, ran-domized trial in patients receiving fractionated courses of radiotherapy to the upper abdomen.[23] Ondansetron (8 mg three times daily) was compared with prochlorperazine (10 mg three times daily). Preliminary analysis of 183 patients again showed an advantage for ondansetron based on the proportion of emesis-free days during treatment (71% vs. 56% with prochlorperazine, P = 0.005).

Preliminary results from two open, pilot studies are available on the use of ondansetron as prophylaxis against emesis produced by total-body ir-radiation and chemotherapy conditioning for bone marrow transplanta-tion.[24] In the first study, ondansetron achieved complete or major control of emesis in 73% of children during cyclophosphamide treatment and in 82% during total body irradiation. Ondansetron was also effective in the second trial, achieving complete or major control during chemotherapy conditioning in 36% to 76% of patients and during total-body irradiation in 74% to 95%.[24]

Granisetron is another 5-HT$_3$ receptor antagonist that has shown the potential to prevent or abolish established chemotherapy-induced nausea and vomiting. Its pharmacodynamic effects provide antiemetic protection for up to 24 hours in patients undergoing chemotherapy. The significant antiemetic effect of this agent in patients undergoing total-body irradiation prompted investigators to explore its use with lower hemibody radiother-apy. Granisetron was recently studied in 22 patients; 13 received 20 mcg/kg and 9 received 40 mcg/kg as an intravenous infusion 1 hour before radio-therapy[25] with a single exposure to the lower half of the body (midline dose of 8 Gy).[25] Nausea and vomiting were completely prevented in 9 of the 13 patients receiving the smaller dose and in 6 of the 9 patients given the larger dose.

Additional studies are planned to compare the effectiveness of grani-setron with that of conventional antiemetic agents. With growing evidence of the effectiveness of 5-HT$_3$ antagonists in patients undergoing radiother-apy, clinical trials are likely to focus on combination antiemetic therapy, including agents such as dexamethasone. The goal is to identify optimal approaches for the prevention or relief of nausea and vomiting.

References

1. Westbrook C, Glaholm J, Barrett A. Vomiting associated with whole body irradiation. *Clin Radiol.* 1987;38:263–266.

2. Harding RK. Prodromal effects of radiation: pathways, models, and protection by antiemetics. *Pharm Ther.* 1988;39:335–345.

3. Hunt EL, Kimeldorf DJ. The humoral factor in radiation-induced motivation. *Radiat Res.* 1967;30:404–419.

4. Carpenter DO, Briggs DB, Knox AP, et al. Peptide-induced emesis in dogs. *Behav Brain Res.* 1984;11:472–474.

5. Wu M, Harding RK, Hugenholtz H, et al. Emetic effects of centrally administered angiotensin II arginine vasopressin and neurotensin in the dog. *Peptides.* 1985;6:173–175.

6. Barnes JH. The physiology and pharmacology of emesis. *Molec Aspects Med.* 1984;7:397–508.

7. Brizzee KR. Effect of localized brain stem lesions and supradiaphragmatic vagotomy on X-irradiation emesis in the monkey. *Am J Physiol.* 1956;187:567–570.

8. Harding RK, Hugenholtz H, Keaney M, et al. Discrete lesions of the area postrema abolish radiation-induced emesis in the dog. *Neurosci Lett.* 1985;53:95–100.

9. Harding RK, Hugenholtz H, Kucharczyk J. Evidence for a high and a low sensitivity receptor site for radiation induced vomiting in the dog. Abstract. 35th Annual Meeting of the Radiation Research Society; 1987:78.

10. Carpenter DO, Briggs DB, Strominger NL. Radiation-induced emesis in the dog: effects of lesions and drugs. *Radiat Res.* 1986;108:307–316.

11. Spitzer TR, Deeg J, Torrisi M, et al. Total body irradiation (TBI) induced emesis is universal after small dose fractions (120cGy) and is not cumulative dose related. Abstract. *Proc Am Soc Clin Oncol.* 1990;9:14.

12. Danjouox CE, Rider WD, Fitzpatrick PJ. The acute radiation syndrome: a memorial to William Michael Court Brown. *Clin Radiol.* 1979;30:581–584.

13. Fytak S, Moertel CG. Management of nausea and vomiting in the cancer patient. *JAMA.* 1981;245;393–396.

14. Herman TS, Einhorn LH, Jones SE. Superiority of nabilone over prochlorperazine as an antiemetic in patients receiving cancer chemotherapy. *N Engl J Med.* 1979;300:1295–1297.

15. Priestman SG, Priestman TJ, Canney PA. A double-blind randomised cross-over comparison of nabilone and metoclopramide in the control of radiation-induced nausea. *Clin Radiol.* 1987;38:1–2.

16. Cunningham D, Forrest GJ, Soukop M, et al. Nabilone and prochlorperazine: a useful combination for emesis induced by cytotoxic drugs. *Br Med J.* 1985;291:864–865.

17. Lucraft HH, Palmer MK. Randomised clinical trial of levonantradol and chlorpromazine in the prevention of radiotherapy-induced vomiting. *Clin Radiol.* 1982;33:621–622.

18. Sokol GH, Greenberg HM, McCarthy S. Radiation induced nausea (RIN): the comparative efficacy of oral metoclopramide (M) versus prochlorperazine (P) and placebo (PL): double blind randomized study. Abstract. *Proc Am Soc Clin Oncol.* 1986;5:248.

19. Gunning SJ, Hagan RM, Tyers BM. Cisplatin induces biochemical and histological changes in the small intestine of the ferret. *Br J Pharmacol.* 1987;90:135P.

20. Andrews PLR, Hawthorn J, Sanger GJ. The effect of abdominal visceral nerve lesions and a novel 5HT-M receptor antagonist on cytotoxic and radiation induced emesis in the ferret. *J Physiol.* 1986;382:47P.

21. Priestman TJ, Roberts JT, Lucraft H. Results of a randomized, double-blind comparative study of ondansetron and metoclopramide in the prevention of nausea and vomiting following high-dose upper abdominal irradiation. *Clin Oncol.* 1990;2:71–75.

22. Collis CH, Priestman TJ, Priestman S. The final assessment of a randomized double-blind comparative study of ondansetron vs. metoclopramide in the prevention of nausea and vomiting following high-dose upper abdominal irradiation. Letter. *Clin Oncol.* 1991;3:241–243.

23. Priestman TJ, Roberts JT, Lucraft H, Upadhyaya BK. Randomized double-blind trial of ondansetron (OND) and prochlorperazine (PCP) in the prevention of radiotherapy (RT) induced emesis. Abstract. *Proc Am Soc Clin Oncol.* 1992;13:1370.

24. Hewitt M, Croockewit S, Abram WP. Ondansetron prophylaxis against emesis produced by total body irradiation and chemotherapy conditioning for bone marrow transplantation. *Eur J Cancer.* 1991; abstract no. 1803.

25. Logue JP, Magee B, Hunter RD. The antiemetic effect of granisetron in lower hemibody radiotherapy. *Clin Oncol.* 1991;3:247–249.

Treatment of Chemotherapy-Induced Emesis

Paul J. Hesketh, MD

Few side effects are as debilitating, distressing to patients, and potentially devastating to the effectiveness of a treatment plan as chemotherapy-induced emesis. Although cancer chemotherapy has produced dramatic responses, fear of its toxic effects can prevent patients from completing curative courses of treatment.[1]

While the emetogenic potential of chemotherapeutic agents has led the public to mistakenly believe that nausea and vomiting are inevitable consequences of such treatment, impressive antiemetic advances during the last decade have begun to change that perception. Discrete emetic problems have been identified, understanding of the physiology of emesis has been improved, effective antiemetic agents have been found (Fig 1), useful doses and schedules for these agents have been established, and, as a result, the ability to prevent emesis has markedly improved.[2] The rapid pace of research in the last 10 years stands in sharp contrast to the lack of progress and relative ineffectiveness of earlier strategies. Before the mid-1970s, there was a paucity of effective antiemetic agents, with phenothiazines constituting the mainstay of emesis management.[3]

Despite the advances, the effectiveness of antiemetic therapy still has significant limitations:

- Nearly one third of patients receiving a cisplatin-based regimen experience emesis within the first 24 hours after treatment.
- The intensely emetogenic preparatory regimens now being used with bone marrow transplantation have created a new population of patients whose emesis control is far from optimal.[3]
- Problems remain with the toxic effects of conventional antiemetic agents, including extrapyramidal reactions to antidopaminergic agents.
- The optimal control of anticipatory and delayed emesis, both of which are still often refractory to antiemetic agents, remains a troublesome problem.

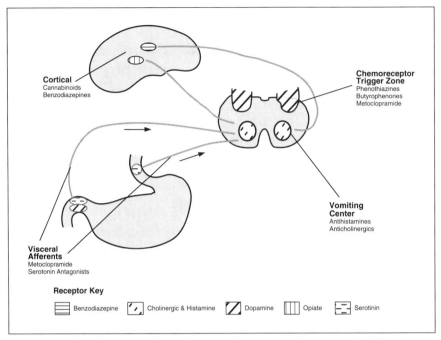

Fig 1. Proposed mechanisms and sites of action of antiemetics. (From Tortorice PV, O'Connell MB. Management of chemotherapy-induced nausea and vomiting. *Pharmacotherapy.* 1990;10:129–145.)

The three major drawbacks of inadequate antiemetic therapy are failure to comply with treatment, patient discomfort, and a variety of medical complications. Estimates vary widely on the percentage of patients who inadequately comply with chemotherapy regimens because of nausea and vomiting, but it may be as high as 25% to 50%. Occasionally, patients have declined potentially curative treatment.[4] The debilitating effects of nausea and vomiting on the personal and social lives of patients lead to a deterioration in their quality of life. Women undergoing monthly adjuvant chemotherapy are sometimes incapacitated for 3 to 4 days and are unable to work during that period. Severe nausea and vomiting also increase the risk for major medical complications, including esophageal tears and dehydration. A less dramatic but more common problem is the prolonged anorexia and malnutrition that compound the frequent cachexia of cancer patients, complicating efforts to administer full dosages of chemotherapy.[4] Depending on the severity and duration of vomiting, major metabolic disturbances, including metabolic alkalosis, and chloride and potassium depletion, may complicate treatment efforts, and these fluid and electrolyte abnormalities must be managed before chemotherapy can continue.

Patients receiving emetogenic chemotherapy may experience three types of emesis, each with distinct patterns:

(1) *Acute-onset emesis,* in which nausea and vomiting are induced within 24 hours after chemotherapy. This is the most widely recognized and studied type of chemotherapy-induced emesis.[5]

(2) *Delayed emesis,* characterized by nausea and vomiting occurring more than 24 hours after chemotherapy administration and continuing for up to 5 days. The precise causes of this phenomenon are still unclear, but symptoms may be related to the action of chemotherapeutic agents (or their metabolites) on the nervous system or gastrointestinal tract.[6] Another possibility is a rebound effect, in which the emetic center or gut is stimulated upon cessation of the receptor-blocking effects of the antiemetics used to treat acute emesis.[6]

(3) *Anticipatory nausea and vomiting* manifests before administration of chemotherapy and may occur in up to 25% of patients. It is probably a conditioned response associated with prior poor antiemetic control during chemotherapy and may be triggered by odors, tastes, or thoughts of chemotherapy. Anticipatory emesis is often refractory to standard antiemetic treatment.

Factors Influencing Emesis

Patient Factors

Age, history of alcohol intake, prior emesis with chemotherapy, and gender are potentially important factors affecting treatment of emesis.[2]

Age. Whether age is directly involved as a factor in controlling emesis remains controversial. It is clear, however, that younger patients have a greater tendency to acute dystonic reactions to antiemetics that act by antagonizing dopamine receptors. As a result, antiemetics such as the substituted benzamides, butyrophenones, and phenothiazines might be more difficult to administer to younger patients. Newer antiemetic agents that block serotonin type 3 receptors may be more useful in younger patients because they do not cause dystonic reactions.[2]

Alcohol intake. Less emesis is encountered in patients with histories of chronic alcohol usage (>100 g/day or five mixed drinks) than in patients who are not heavy drinkers.

Poor emetic control in past. Patients with a history of poor emetic control are predisposed to unsatisfactory treatment. It is unclear whether such reactions are related to conditioned anticipatory emesis.

Gender. Although there is growing evidence that it is more difficult to control emesis in women than in men, this issue is still controversial. Its

125

resolution is complicated by the fact that women in antiemetic studies tend to be receiving two or more emetogenic agents and are less likely to have had histories of heavy alcohol use. Large trials are needed before questions surrounding the role of gender are answered.[2]

Treatment Factors

Categorizing the emetic potential of 40 antineoplastic drugs, a recent report calls attention to important considerations in the selection of appropriate antiemetic agents.[5] The highly emetogenic drugs such as cisplatin and mechlorethamine, for example, produce nausea and vomiting in more than 90% of patients receiving inadequate antiemetic therapy (Table 1). Drugs considered to be moderately emetogenic, such as cyclophosphamide, produce such complications in 30% to 90%. Among the most important factors in determining the emetogenic potential of antineoplastic drugs are the following:

- The frequency of chemotherapy-induced emesis with combination regimens is not always predictable, but it generally is comparable to that of the most emetogenic drug administered.
- The intensity of emesis is usually related to the dose and course of chemotherapy treatment. For example, low doses of cisplatin tend to be better tolerated than larger doses.
- Although the particular chemotherapeutic agent largely determines the duration of emesis, most drugs are emetogenic for about 12 to 24 hours after administration. A notable exception, however, is cisplatin.

Both the drug dose and the route of administration can affect the incidence of nausea and vomiting.[2] Most moderate to highly emetogenic chemotherapeutic agents will induce emesis within 1 to 2 hours after the start of treatment in the absence of effective antiemetics. But when cyclophosphamide is administered intravenously in high doses, the onset of emesis is often delayed until 9 to 18 hours after chemotherapy. The importance of rate and route of chemotherapy and its impact on emetic onset, intensity, and duration are illustrated with plicamycin and cytarabine. In both cases, onset of severe emesis is earlier with rapid administration than with slower infusion rates. Different patterns of emesis are also found when chemotherapy is administered via continuous infusion compared with bolus injection. With continuous infusion, nausea and vomiting usually peak within the first day of treatment and gradually diminish, leaving the patient almost symptom free by the end of the regimen.[5]

The Pathophysiology of Chemotherapy-Induced Emesis

Emesis comprises a complex sequence of events in which the coordinated activation of the nervous, gastrointestinal, respiratory, and cardiovascular

Table 1. Relative Emetic Potential of Antineoplastic Drugs

High (> 90%)	Moderately High (60–90%)	Moderate (30–60%)	Moderately Low (10–30%)	Low (<10%)
Cisplatin	Semustine	5-Fluorouracil	Bleomycin	Busulfan
Dacarbazine	Carmustine	Doxorubicin	Hydroxyurea	Chlorambucil
Mechlorethamine	Lomustine	Daunorubicin	Melphalan	6-Thioguanine
Streptozotocin	Cyclophosphamide	L-Asparaginase	Etoposide	Vincristine
Cytarabine*	Actinomycin-D	Mitomycin-C	Teniposide	Estrogens
	Mithramycin	5-Azacytidine	Cytarabine[†]	Progestins
	Procarbazine	Hexamethylmelamine	6-Mercaptopurine	Corticosteroids
	Methotrexate[†]		Methotrexate[§]	Androgens
			Thiotepa	
			Vinblastine	

*Only with "high-dose" therapy (> 500 mg/m2).
[†]Doses > 200 mg/m^2.
[‡]Standard dose.
[§]Low dose.

From Craig JB, Powell BL. The management of nausea and vomiting in clinical oncology. *Am J Med Sci.* 1987;293:34–44.

systems ultimately leads to expulsion of gastric contents.[7,8] The emetic response may have evolved as a defense mechanism to enable elimination of toxic substances from the gastrointestinal tract.[9]

Emesis encompasses three processes—nausea, retching, and vomiting—which are often but not always activated in sequential fashion.[7,8,10] Usually a precursor to retching and vomiting, nausea can be prolonged, either before or after vomiting, and may occur in the absence of vomiting. It is often accompanied by prodromal signs, such as salivation, pupillary dilatation, tachypnea, and tachycardia, which indicate overactivity of the autonomic nervous system. Spontaneous contractile activity of the stomach decreases with the onset of nausea. Prior to vomiting, the proximal stomach relaxes, and the small intestine is evacuated by retrograde peristaltic contractions. Contraction of the internal intercostal muscles out of phase with other respiratory muscles results in retching. The periesophageal portion of the diaphragm then relaxes, and subsequent contraction of the external intercostals, diaphragm, and abdominal muscles results in the expulsion of gastric contents. Unlike nausea, which depends on autonomic activity, retching and vomiting are controlled by the somatic nervous system (Fig 2).

Models of the Emetic Response

Studies approximately 40 years ago helped shape current concepts about the emetic response. Based on ablation and electrical stimulation experiments, primarily in cats and dogs, Borison and Wang[11] proposed that two critical and distinct sites in the brainstem control emesis. One site serves as an entry point for emetogenic humoral substances, and the other coordinates motor mechanisms of emesis. Labelled the "vomiting center," the latter site is located in the lateral reticular formation of the medulla and serves as the final common pathway through which afferent stimuli activate the emetic reflex. The vomiting center lies adjacent to structures that help coordinate vomiting, including the respiratory, vasomotor, and salivary centers and eighth and tenth cranial nerves. Another important medullary structure is the chemoreceptor trigger zone (CTZ), situated in the area postrema, a circumventricular structure at the caudal aspect of the fourth ventricle. Outside the blood-brain barrier, the CTZ is accessible to humoral emetic stimuli borne by blood or cerebrospinal fluid. Although it cannot independently initiate emesis, it can activate the vomiting center.

Three other major sources of afferent input to the emetic center include the vestibular apparatus that plays a role in motion sickness, the pharynx and gastrointestinal tract, and higher brainstem and cortical structures. Afferent input from the pharynx and gastrointestinal tract travels to the vomiting center predominantly via the vagus nerve, with some input from splanchnic nerves. Electrical stimulation of supramedullary structures (cerebral cortex, hypothalamus, and thalamus) can also evoke emesis and is critical for anticipatory emesis.

Although these basic concepts have remained essentially the same for 40 years, new observations have reshaped our understanding of emesis. For example, it is now appreciated that an anatomically distinct vomiting center cannot be defined. Recent studies suggest that the complex motor activity in emesis is coordinated by a control pattern generator located in the nucleus tractus solitarius.

In addition to the pivotal role of the area postrema in humorally mediated emesis, other receptors for chemically induced emesis have been recognized. Animal models indicate that abolition of the area postrema eliminates an emetic response, suggesting that the area postrema may be the critical site of action for that emetic stimulus. This concept is classically illustrated by abolition of the emetic response to apomorphine with the

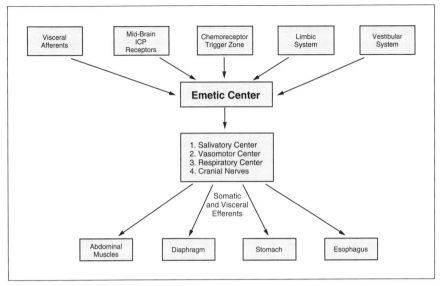

Fig 2. Reflex pathways of vomiting. Vomiting can be triggered by afferent impulses to the emetic center from the chemoreceptor trigger zone, vestibular apparatus, midbrain, limbic system, or periphery (pharynx and gastrointestinal tract). Afferent impulses are integrated by the emetic center. Vomiting results from output to the neighboring medullary control centers, with subsequent stimulation of somatic and visceral efferent impulses to the effector organs. (From Siegel L, Longo D. The control of chemotherapy-induced emesis. *Ann Intern Med.* 1981;95:353.)

experimental destruction of the area postrema.[12] Apomorphine appears to induce emesis by binding to dopamine receptors in the area postrema. Other mechanisms may be involved with different forms of emetic stimuli. For example, the area postrema is an important terminus for abdominal vagal afferents,[13] which exert significant influences on it.[14] Consequently, an emetic stimulus may primarily increase vagal afferent transmission, with a secondary, vagally mediated effect on the area postrema.

Thus, although experimental destruction of the area postrema may mute the emetic effect of a stimulus, the area postrema may not be the primary site but simply part of the neural pathway for that emetic stimulus. However, ablation of the area postrema would eliminate emesis if an emetic stimulus triggered the release from the gut of an emetic substance that could activate the area postrema through blood-borne transmission.[10]

Neurotransmitters

The focus of investigations on neurochemical mechanisms underlying emesis has broadened from central nervous system structures—where at least 30 distinct neurochemicals have been found—to include the role of neuroactive substances in peripherally mediated emesis. An association has emerged between the emetic response and various types of neurotransmitter receptors, contributing to speculation that the neurotransmitters involved in chemotherapy-induced emesis include dopamine, histamine, acetylcholine, endogenous opiates, and serotonin.[10,15–18]

Although many studies have explored the role of these compounds in the pathophysiology of chemotherapy-induced emesis and the potential role of various antagonists, information is still lacking on the precise mechanisms by which cytotoxic agents stimulate the emetic response. It may be that chemotherapy inactivates enzymes essential for the breakdown of neurotransmitters,[19] and emesis results when the neurotransmitter exceeds a certain concentration. Other investigators speculate that metabolites of chemotherapeutic agents or products of chemotherapy-damaged cells interact with the area postrema. Still other theories propose that chemotherapy may affect taste perception,[20] the vestibular system,[21] cerebral cortex and other supramedullary loci,[18] and peripheral receptors in the pharynx and upper gastrointestinal tract.[22]

Treatment of Acute-Onset Emesis

Progress in antiemetic control has been greatest in the management of acute-onset emesis, which has been more intensively studied than either delayed or anticipatory nausea and vomiting. Several classes of agents have been used.

Dopaminergic Antagonists
- **Phenothiazines.** Phenothiazines were the first family of agents demonstrated to have significant antiemetic activity. In addition to their dopamine receptor blockade, phenothiazines also may be effective because of their anticholinergic activity in the vomiting and vestibular centers of the brain.[5] The phenothiazines showing the most potent antiemetic activity include prochlorperazine, thiethylperazine, and perphenazine.

Despite their effectiveness with mildly emetogenic chemotherapy, the phenothiazines have a limited role in controlling chemotherapy-induced emesis with the more emetogenic regimens, unless used in high doses or combined with other antiemetics.[23] As a class, the phenothiazines are well tolerated; common side effects include sedation, anticholinergic effects, and anti-alpha-adrenergic effects.
- **Butyrophenones.** Another group of dopaminergic antagonists are the butyrophenones, which include haloperidol and droperidol. Their stronger central dopaminergic blockade offers advantages over phenothiazines.[5] Although antiemetic trials have shown a pattern of variable re-

sponse with this drug class, the butyrophenones are considered beneficial for use with moderately severe emetogenic chemotherapy. The major side effect associated with their use is sedation; extrapyramidal reactions can occur but are less frequent than with the phenothiazines.[23]

Substituted Benzamides

Metoclopramide. Numerous studies have focused on the use of metoclopramide, which until recently was the most commonly used antiemetic and the most effective of the substituted benzamides.[2] Metoclopramide's antiemetic activity may result from several of its actions: blocking dopaminergic stimulation of the CTZ, increasing gastric motility, alleviating stasis, and at high doses, antagonizing serotonin receptors centrally or in the gastrointestinal tract. The drug is well absorbed with onset of action 20 to 30 minutes after oral administration, and parenteral doses are effective within 1 to 3 minutes.[23]

Early studies employing metoclopramide at standard doses (0.15 mg/kg to 0.30 mg/kg) administered intravenously (IV) failed to note any significant efficacy in controlling chemotherapy-induced emesis. Gralla and others were the first to note the efficacy of using higher doses (1 mg/kg) in the prevention of cisplatin-induced emesis.[24] When used as a single agent, IV high-dose (1 to 3 mg/kg) metoclopramide has been shown to be superior to placebo, tetrahydrocannabinol, dexamethasone, prochlorperazine, and haloperidol for cisplatin-induced emesis, completely preventing vomiting in about 40% of patients.

Although a true dose-response relationship for metoclopramide has not been established,[23] there has been considerable study of high doses of the drug in cisplatin-induced emesis. A response rate of 75% has been demonstrated with doses greater than 1.75 mg/kg, compared with 56% when the drug is used at lower doses.[23] Major side effects of metoclopramide include sedation, diarrhea, and extrapyramidal symptoms.

Investigations have explored whether continuous IV infusion of metoclopramide will improve the drug's safety and efficacy for high-dose therapy and to make it more cost effective. There is no clear cut evidence, however, that such an approach is superior to IV bolus therapy. Recent studies[23] have shown that a high dose of metoclopramide (3 mg/kg) given as a single dose may be more advantageous. The rationale behind this strategy is based on these points: (1) a single dose of metoclopramide given prior to chemotherapy would be more convenient and economical; (2) a high peak level of metoclopramide would be assured, and a therapeutic level would likely be maintained throughout the period of potential emesis; and (3) in addition to the antidopaminergic effects, such high levels would probably block 5-HT$_3$ receptors as well.[2]

Cannabinoids

First observed in anecdotal reports, the effectiveness of tetrahydrocannabinol (THC) in relieving chemotherapy-induced emesis has been evaluated in numerous trials. Conflicting results raise questions about the extent to which this drug class is effective and to what extent it can be used in different patient populations. Two cannabinoids, dronabinol and nabilone, are available for chemotherapy-induced emesis. The mechanism of action of these agents is still unclear, but it may be related to their effects on opiate receptors and cortical and/or brainstem areas of the brain. Randomized trials have demonstrated that THC is more effective than placebo, prochlorperazine, low-dose metoclopramide, and haloperidol when tested against low-to-moderate emetogenic agents. However, THC has not been shown to be as effective as high-dose metoclopramide. The selection of a cannabinoid is tempered by its side effects, which have led patients to prefer a less effective antiemetic. It appears that the addition of a phenothiazine can limit the incidence of adverse effects with THC. The most significant central nervous system side effects associated with THC are mood changes, memory loss, problems with motor coordination, altered sensorium, hallucinations, euphoria, relaxation, and hunger.[5] Cannabinoids may be useful in combination with other antiemetics, but their side effects and potential for abuse will probably limit their administration to younger patients.

Corticosteroids

Another useful class of agents are the corticosteroids. Although several theories have been proposed to explain their mechanism of action, it is still unclear how corticosteroids like dexamethasone exert their antiemetic effect. Among the more popular explanations are inhibition of prostaglandin synthesis and a possible role in mood elevation, increased appetite, and an induced sense of well-being. Studies have confirmed the efficacy of dexamethasone when used in a dose range of 4 mg to 20 mg.[25] One trial indicated that a single dose of dexamethasone given 30 minutes before cisplatin was as effective as a two- or three-dose schedule started hours before chemotherapy. Toxicity has generally been mild with short courses of dexamethasone or methylprednisolone, and these agents apparently do not compromise the efficacy of chemotherapy. The consensus seems to be that dexamethasone is best used as a single agent with moderately emetogenic chemotherapy; it is less effective against highly emetogenic regimens, although it is a useful addition to combination antiemetic regimens.[25]

Benzodiazepines

Benzodiazepines as single agents have very limited antiemetic efficacy, but are often useful additions to antiemetic regimens.[2] Lorazepam, for example, is well accepted by patients, and it is markedly effective in reducing akathisia and anxiety. These agents may be working in this setting by relieving anxiety-related distress and depression as well as inhibiting of the vomiting center. These effects also may support the use of lorazepam for anticipatory emesis. Doses of 1 to 1.5 mg/m^2 have been used effectively and can be repeated every 4 hours.[9] Midazolam, a parenteral benzodiazepine with a rapid onset and ultra-short half-life, may be an alternative to lorazepam for chemotherapy-induced emesis,[5] principally because its sedative effect is less than that of lorazepam. Experience with benzodiazepines suggests that they will continue to be used as adjuncts for antiemetic regimens because of their wide patient acceptance, and minimal toxicity.[5]

Serotonin Antagonists

Despite significant advances in antiemetic treatment over the last decade, a considerable proportion of patients still experience emesis after chemotherapy. In addition, side effects, including sedation, extrapyradimal effects, and dystonic reactions, remain fundamental problems. Selective serotonin antagonists are a genuinely new class of agents capable of addressing such issues and expanding awareness of basic physiologic and pathophysiologic pathways. Serotonin is a ubiquitous substance associated with processes as diverse as migraine headache and control of appetite and mood.[1] The serotonin type 3 receptor, 5-hydroxytryptamine$_3$ (5-HT$_3$), which is found in both the gastrointestinal tract and the central nervous system, appears to be a principal mediator of the emetic reflex.

Serendipitously, investigations with metoclopramide, the prototypical antidopaminergic agent, set the stage for development of new concepts about pathways of chemotherapy-induced emesis. Unlike the other dopamine D2 receptor antagonists, high-dose metoclopramide was effective in reducing emesis associated with cisplatin, leading to speculation that an unexplored antiemetic mechanism was involved. Indeed, early investigators had demonstrated that metoclopramide, in addition to its capacity for dopaminergic antagonism, was also a weak 5-HT$_3$ antagonist. This provided a rationale for the subsequent development and study of selective 5-HT$_3$ antagonists, which were devoid of antidopaminergic effects, as antiemetics. Recent studies have confirmed the clinical utility of selective 5-HT$_3$ antagonists as entiemetics.[3] The precise mechanisms by which the 5-HT$_3$ antagonists act remain incompletely defined. One clue may be provided by studying the means by which cisplatin is able to induce emesis.

Serotonin tends to be concentrated in the gastrointestinal tract, primarily within the enterochromaffin cells of the mucosal layer. Levels of serotonin within the mucosa are increased when cisplatin damages the epithelium of the small intestine. An abundance of 5-HT$_3$ receptors can be found on vagal afferents and neurons within the gastrointestinal tract. Serotonin may bind to 5-HT$_3$ receptors on visceral afferents that run from the gut to the emetic center and area postrema. The latter area may operate as a relay between visceral afferents and the emetic center.[3] Disruption of afferent transmission at this level by 5-HT$_3$ receptor antagonists appears to be effective in preventing chemotherapy-induced emesis.

A number of selective serotonin antagonists have been studied for their potential clinical utility in preventing chemotherapy-induced emesis. The most extensively evaluated agents to date have been ondansetron and granisetron.

Ondansetron

Early studies in patients receiving cisplatin-based chemotherapy demonstrated significant antiemetic activity for ondansetron over a wide dose range (0.04 mg/kg to 0.48 mg/kg in three divided doses, IV) and established its safety and tolerability.[3] A variety of dosing schedules have been tested and similar response rates have been obtained with intermittent dosing at 2-, 4-, 6-, or 8-hour intervals.[3] Recently a large double-blind randomized trial compared the currently approved dose and schedule (0.15 mg/kg IV every 4 hours X 3 doses) of ondansetron with two fixed single-dose regimens (8 mg and 32 mg) in chemotherapy-naive patients receiving cisplatin chemotherapy. The 32 mg single dose was more effective than the 8 mg single dose and at least as effective as the standard 3-dose regimen in preventing acute cisplatin-induced emesis.[26]

Three randomized single-agent comparisons of ondansetron and high-dose metoclopramide have consistently noted either comparable or superior activity for ondansetron in preventing acute cisplatin-induced emesis. In addition, ondansetron was better tolerated than metoclopramide in the latter trials (Figs 3 and 4).[3]

An important issue from a clinical standpoint is the ability of an antiemetic agent to maintain high efficacy with repeated cisplatin cycles over several months. In this setting, preliminary data from a retrospective analysis by Gandara et al[27] indicate that approximately 80% of those patients with a major response during the initial cycle, continued to respond during 2 to 8 additional cycles of cisplatin therapy. Encouraging antiemetic results have also been obtained when ondansetron was used with non-ciplastin chemotherapy, for breast cancer patients who received cyclophosphamide, fluorouracil, and doxorubicin.[28]

Granisetron

Granisetron is another extremely potent 5-HT$_3$ antagonist developed specifically as an antiemetic.[3] The drug has a prolonged half-life of approximately 8 to 10 hours, suggesting that a single IV dose of 40 µg/kg might be

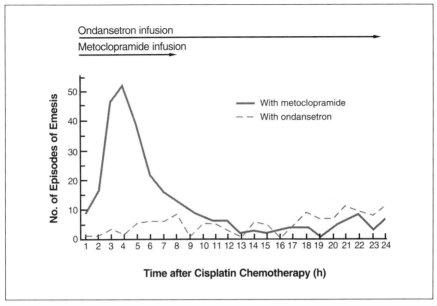

Fig 3. Episodes of emesis during the 24 hours after cisplatin administration in patients given ondansetron or metoclopramide. (From Marty M, et al. Comparison of the 5-hydroxytryptamine$_3$ (serotonin) antagonist ondansetron (GR38032F) with high-dose metoclopramide in the control of cisplatin-induced emesis. *N Engl J Med.* 1990;322:816−821.)

effective in preventing chemotherapy-induced emesis. When two doses of granisetron, 40 μg/kg and 160 μg/kg, were compared the difference in efficacy, 69% vs. 73% complete protection, was not significant and 89% of patients required only one dose.[29]

In a trial that compared a single dose of granisetron with the combination of metoclopramide, dexamethasone, and diphenhydramine,[29] superior and complete control was achieved with granisetron during the first 6 hours. However, emesis and nausea were significantly more frequent at 18 hours to 24 hours in granisetron-treated patients.[30] Yet, in another study comparing a single dose of granisetron, 40 mg/kg, with a combination of high-dose metoclopramide and dexamethasone in patients receiving cisplatin, the antiemetic efficacy between the two treatment arms was comparable.[31]

Other Selective 5-HT$_3$ Antagonists

A host of other selective 5-HT$_3$ antagonists, such as ICS 205−930, and MDL 73147 EF are in various stages of clinical development.[3] A number of comparative studies are underway attempting to determine whether significant differences in efficacy exist among these agents.

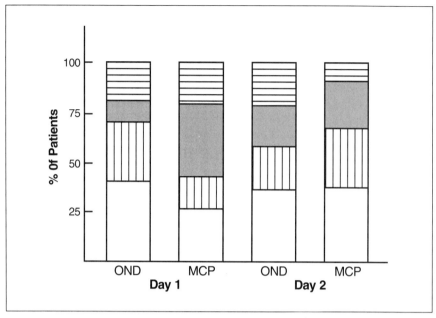

Fig 4. Control of emesis during the acute (day 1) and delayed (days 2 through 6) phases. Open boxes indicate a complete response; vertical hatched boxes indicate a major response; stippled boxes indicate a minor response; horizontal hatched boxes indicate failure; OND = ondansetron; MCP = metoclopramide. On day 1, n = 95 and $P \leq 0.001$. On days 2 through 6, n = 79 and $P = 0.212$. (From De Mulder PHM, Seynaeve C, Vermorkeu JB, et al. Ondansetron compared with high-dose metoclopramide in prophylaxis of acute and delayed cisplatin-induced nausea and vomiting. *Ann Intern Med.* 1990;113:834–840.)

Combination Therapy

With studies pointing toward multiple mechanisms for chemotherapy-induced emesis, involving stimulus of several central and peripheral emetic receptors, the rationale for combinations of agents, has grown stronger. The rationale is straightforward and relatively simple: The method of eliminating nausea and vomiting is to block all likely emetic stimuli by combining antiemetics with different mechanisms of action. Some combinations use smaller or fewer doses of effective yet toxic antiemetics; others incorporate adjunctive drugs to treat or prevent adverse effects of antiemetics; other combinations are based on both approaches.[5]

Dexamethasone is probably the most favored agent in such strategies.[5] This drug has been extensively studied in combination with high-dose metoclopramide for cisplatin-induced emesis, and substantial evidence indicates that the combination achieves more complete responses than metoclopramide alone. A three-drug regimen—dexamethasone, metoclopramide, and diphenhydramine—has also been used, with minor improvement inantiemetic response over the metoclopramide-dexamethasone combination, but significantly fewer acute dystonic reactions. As an alternative strategy, transdermal scopolamine has been added to dexamethasone and metoclopramide, reportedly providing significantly more emetic protection.

The success achieved by adding dexamethasone to metoclopramide prompted Italian researchers to study the effectiveness of dexamethasone plus ondansetron.[32] The rate of complete protection from emesis was significantly higher with the combination of ondansetron and dexamethasone than with ondansetron alone, 91% vs. 64%.

In a trend toward more intensive combination regimens, several studies have evaluated the use of four or five drugs for protection against emesis associated with high-dose cisplatin.[5] Oral and parenteral doses of metoclopramide, dexamethasone, diphenhydramine, triethylperazine, and diazepam have been used. It is unclear whether such regimens are superior to combinations employing fewer agents.

A combination of cannabinoids and phenothiazines may improve cannabinoid antiemetic activity while limiting the central nervous system effects associated with THC.[5] Another regimen generating some interest entails the use of a cannabinoid and dexamethasone, which is believed to increase antiemetic efficacy and decrease adverse reactions such as postural hypotension and psychoactive changes.

Several other agents, including lorazepam, have been the focus of premedication drug combination strategies to improve antiemetic efficacy. Lorazepam acts mainly on the cerebral cortex, limbic system, and brain stem reticular formation to induce anxiolysis and sedation, antegrade amnesia, and a dampened response of the vomiting center to a variety of afferent stimuli. In one study[33] 85 patients treated with cisplation were evaluated after randomization to lorazepam, oxazepam, or methylprednisolone. Lorazepam significantly reduced the number of patients with the most severe degrees of vomiting. The duration of vomiting was also reduced significantly after the first 48 hours postchemotherapy in the lorazepam group compared with the methylprednisolone group. Although 10% to 15% of patients in this study found the sedation and amnesia associated with the drug undesirable and even distressing at times,[33] lorazepam appears to have value in combination regimens for the treatment of cisplatin-induced emesis.

Delayed Emesis

As new strategies for treating acute-onset emesis demonstrate improved efficacy, the focus is shifting toward delayed emesis, which has been less studied but remains a major problem. Delayed emesis is defined as nausea or vomiting beginning 24 hours or more after chemotherapy administration.[2] Delayed emesis is generally less severe than the acute form, but it may cause significant difficulties with hydration and nutrition and contribute to a lowered activity level.[2]

The majority of patients treated with cisplatin at doses greater than 100 mg/m^2 experience some degree of delayed emesis. Symptoms usually occur between 1 and 5 days after treatment, with the greatest risk between 2 and 3 days.[5] Because many antiemetic regimens are administered only on the day of chemotherapy, patients at risk for delayed emesis may be unprotected during a vulnerable time.

Little is known about the mechanisms of delayed emesis. Symptoms may be related to the action of chemotherapeutic agents (or their metabolites) on the nervous system or gastrointestinal tract.[6] Another possibility is a "rebound effect," in which the emetic center or gut is stimulated when the receptor-blocking effects of the antiemetics used to treat acute emesis abate.[6]

One of the keys to controlling delayed emesis appears to lie in the effectiveness of treatment during the initial 24 hours, according to results in 86 patients who were treated with cisplatin for the first time.[6] On the day of cisplatin treatment, all received IV metoclopramide (3 mg/kg for two doses) plus IV dexamethasone (20 mg) with either diphenhydramine (50 mg) or lorazepam (1.0 mg/m^2 to 1.5 mg/m^2). The incidence of delayed nausea and emesis peaked between 48 and 72 hours after cisplatin administration. Patients who had no emesis during the initial 24 hours after cisplatin treatment were less likely to experience delayed emesis.

Based on this information, Kris et al[33] prospectively studied the safety and effectiveness of combination therapy in controlling delayed vomiting in 91 patients receiving cisplatin. They were randomized to one of three treatment regimens: placebo; oral dexamethasone (8 mg twice daily for 2 days, then 4 mg twice daily for 2 days); or the combination of oral metoclopramide (0.5 mg/kg four times daily for 4 days) plus oral dexamethasone (administered as above). With the combination, 48% of patients experienced delayed vomiting, significantly better results than the 65% incidence of delayed emesis after dexamethasone alone and the 89% with placebo.[34]

Although the role of 5-HT$_3$ antagonists in the prevention of delayed emesis remains to be defined, some indication of the potential benefit of this class of agents was evident in a study by Gandara et al.[35] Their study suggested that ondansetron may be more effective than placebo in the prevention of emesis occurring 1 to 4 days after high-dose cisplatin treatment. The antiemetic effect was most apparent on the third day, when 21 of 27 patients had a complete response to ondansetron (compared to 7 of 18 given placebo). Further studies are needed before 5-HT$_3$ antagonists can be routinely employed for delayed emesis.

Anticipatory Emesis

Refractory to standard antiemetic therapy, anticipatory emesis is relatively uncommon but remains one of the toughest challenges associated with administration of chemotherapy. Anticipatory emesis is defined as nausea or vomiting, often beginning before the administration of chemotherapy, in patients with poor control of emesis during past chemotherapy treatment. Documenting a prevalence of the syndrome in 33% of 121 patients, Johns Hopkins researchers found that the length of postchemotherapy nausea was significantly related to the presence of anticipatory symptoms.[36] Yet the symptoms were typically mild and generally well managed in this series, in contrast to the widely held clinical impression that anticipatory nausea and vomiting often stand in the way of successful completion of chemotherapy.

Criteria for identifying the patient at high risk for anticipatory vomiting appeared in a report by Morrow,[37] who proposed variables that significantly correlated with development of this emesis. The criteria included the following: less than 50 years of age; nausea or vomiting described by the patient as moderate, severe, or intolerable; susceptibility to motion sickness; and the sensation of sweating or feeling "hot all over"; nausea and vomiting after the last chemotherapy session; sweating after the last chemotherapy session; and generalized weakness after the last chemotherapy session. If four or more of these characteristics were present, the probability was at least 80% that the patient would develop anticipatory vomiting.

Despite the generally disappointing results with pharmacologic treatment, behavioral modification and systemic relaxation may have value in the management of anticipatory emesis. Hypnosis, progressive muscle relaxation, systemic desensitization, biofeedback monitoring, and mind diversion with guided mental imagery have been shown to be of benefit. The most effective approach, however, remains pharmacologic—management of nausea and emesis during the initial course of emesis-producing chemotherapy. Adjunctive pharmacologic treatment with lorazepam and/or behavioral therapy should be given in addition to intensified antiemetic therapy for those at high risk.

Conclusion

Inadequate prevention and treatment of chemotherapy-induced emesis are still substantial problems, resulting in patient discomfort, medical complications, and, occasionally, poor compliance with treatment. However, improved understanding of the pathophysiology of chemotherapy-induced emesis has led to the development of more appropriate and effective antiemetic treatment. Recognition of the value of combination antiemetic therapy has been a major step forward.

Another exciting development has been the identification of a new class of agents, the serotonin antagonists. These agents appear to have efficacy comparable or superior to that of conventional antiemetics with fewer unfavorable side effects. Future studies should focus on combination regimens incorporating serotonin antagonists and should seek more effective means of controlling delayed emesis.

References

1. Grunberg SM. Making chemotherapy easier. *N Engl J Med.* 1990;322:846–848.
2. Gralla RJ. Controlling emesis in patients receiving cancer chemotherapy. *Rec Results Cancer Res.* 1991;121:68–85.
3. Hesketh PJ, Gandara DR. Serotonin antagonists: a new class of antiemetic agents. *J Natl Cancer Inst.* 1991;83:613–620.
4. Laszlo J. Nausea and vomiting as major complications of cancer chemotherapy. *Drugs.* 1983;25(suppl 1):1–7.
5. Tortorice PV, O'Connell MB. Management of chemotherapy-induced nausea and vomiting. *Pharmacotherapy.* 1990;10:129–145.
6. Kris MG, Gralla RJ, Clark RA, et al. Incidence, course, and severity of delayed nausea and vomiting following the administration of high-dose cisplatin. *J Clin Oncol.* 1985;3:1379–1384.
7. McCarthy LE, Borison HL. Respiratory mechanics of vomiting in decerebrate cats. *Am J Physiol.* 1974;226:738–743.
8. Brizee KR. Mechanics of vomiting: a minireview. *Can J Physiol Pharmacol.* 1990;68:221–229.
9. Davis CJ, Harding RR, Leslie RA, et al. The organization of vomiting as a protective reflex. In: Davis CJ, Lake-Bakaar GV, Grahame-Smith DG, eds. *Nausea and Vomiting: Mechanisms and Treatment.* Berlin, Germany: Springer-Verlag; 1986:65–75.
10. Andrews PLR, Rapeport WG, Sanger GJ. Neuropharmacology of emesis induced by anti-cancer therapy. *TIPS.* 1988;9:334–341.
11. Borison HL, Wang SC. Physiology and pharmacology of vomiting. *Pharmacol Rev.* 1953;5:193–230.
12. Wang SC, Borison HL. A new concept in the organization of the central emetic mechanism: recent studies on the sites of action of apomorphine, copper sulfate and cardiac glycosides. *Gastroenterology.* 1952;22:1–12.
13. Leslie RA. Neuroactive substances in the dorsal vagal complex of the medulla oblongata: nucleus of the tractus solitarius, area postrema and dorsal motor nucleus of the vagus. *Neurochem Int.* 1985;7:191–211.
14. Andrews PLR, Davis CJ, Bingham S, et al. The abdominal visceral innervation and the emetic reflex: pathways, pharmacology, and plasticity. *Can J Physiol Pharmacol.* 1990;68:325–345.
15. Leslie RA, Shah Y, Thejomayen M, et al. The neuropharmacology of emesis: the role of receptors in neuromodulation of nausea and vomiting. *Can J Physiol Pharmacol.* 1990;68:279–288.
16. Stewart DJ. Cancer therapy, vomiting, and antiemetics. *Can J Physiol Pharmacol.* 1990;68:304–313.
17. Peroutka SJ, Synder SH. Antiemetics: neurotransmitter receptor binding predicts therapeutic action. *Lancet.* 1982;1:658–659.
18. Borison HL, McCarthy LE. Neuropharmacology of chemotherapy-induced emesis. *Drugs.* 1983;25(suppl):8–17.

19. Harris AL, Cantwell BMJ. Mechanisms and treatment of cytotoxic-induced nausea and vomiting. In: Davis CJ, Lake-Bakaar GV, Grahame-Smith DG, eds. *Nausea and Vomiting: Mechanisms and Treatment.* Berlin, Germany: Springer-Verlag; 1986:78–93.

20. Fetting JH, Wilcox PM, Sheidler VR, et al. Tastes associated with parenteral chemotherapy for breast cancer. *Cancer Treat Rep.* 1985;69:1249–1251.

21. Morrow GR. The effect of a susceptibility to motion sickness on the side effects of cancer chemotherapy. *Cancer.* 1985;55:2766–2770.

22. Miner WE, Sanger GJ, Turner DH. Evidence that 5-hydroxytryptamine-3 receptors mediate cytotoxic drug and radiation-invoked emesis. *Br J Cancer.* 1987;56:159.

23. Craig JB, Powell BL. The management of nausea and vomiting in clinical oncology. *Am J Med Sci.* 1987;293:34–44.

24. Gralla R, Itri L, Pisko S, et al. Antiemetic efficacy of high dose metoclopramide: randomized trials with placebo and prochlorperazine in patients with chemotherapy-induced vomiting. *N Engl J Med.* 1981;305:905–909.

25. Gralla RJ, Tyson LB, Kris MG, et al. The management of chemotherapy-induced nausea and vomiting. *Med Clin N Am.* 1987;71:289–301.

26. Beck TM, Hesketh PJ, Madujewicz S, et al. A stratified, randomized, double-blind comparison of intravenous ondansetron administered as a multiple dose regimen versus two single dose regimens, in the prevention of cisplatin-induced nausea and vomiting. *J Clin Oncol.* 1992;10:1969–1975.

27. Gandara DR, Werner K, Perez EA, et al. Effectiveness of retreatment with GR-38032F in control of cisplatin-induced nausea and vomiting. *Eur Conf Clin Oncol.* 1989;5:P-0525.

28. Franschini G, Esparza L, Ciociola A, et al. Evaluation of three oral dosages of ondansetron (GR38032F) in the prevention of emesis associated with doxorubicin-cyclophosphamide chemotherapy. *Proc Am Soc Clin Oncol.* 1990;9:328.

29. Tabona MV. Granisetron (G) in the prevention of cytostatic-induced emesis. *Proc Am Soc Clin Oncol.* 1990;9:319.

30. Venner P. Granisetron for high-dose cisplatin (HDCP)-induced emesis: a randomized double-blind study. *Proc Am Soc Clin Oncol.* 1990;9:320.

31. Chevallier B. Efficacy and safety of granisetron compared with high-dose metoclopramide plus dexamethasone in patients receiving high-dose cisplatin in a single-blind study. *Eur J Cancer.* 1990;26:S33-S36.

32. Roila F, Tonato M, Cognetti F, et al. Prevention of cisplatin-induced emesis: a double-blind multicenter randomized crossover study comparing ondansetron and ondansetron plus dexamethasone. *J Clin Oncol.* 1991;9:675–678.

33. Kearsley JH, Williams AM, Fiumara B. Antiemetic superiority of lorazepam over oxazepam and methylprednisolone as premedicants for patients receiving cisplatin-containing chemotherapy. *Cancer.* 1989;64:1595–1599.

34. Kris M, Gralla RJ, Tyson LB, et al. Controlling delayed vomiting: double-blind, randomized trial comparing placebo, dexamethasone alone, and metoclopramide plus dexamethasone in patients receiving cisplatin. *J Clin Oncol.* 1989;7:108–114.

35. Gandara DR, Harvey WH, Monoghan GG, et al. Efficacy of ondansetron in the prevention of delayed emesis following high-dose cisplatin (DDP). *Proc Am Soc Clin Oncol.* 1990;9:328.

36. Stefanek ME, Sheidler VR, Fetting JH. Anticipatory nausea and vomiting: does it remain a significant clinical problem? *Cancer.* 1988;62:2654–2657.

37. Morrow G. Clinical characteristics associated with the development of anticipatory nausea and vomiting in cancer patients undergoing chemotherapy treatment. *J Clin Oncol.* 1984;2:1170–1176.

Nausea or Vomiting Associated with Poisoning or Drug Overdose

Susan Kim, PharmD, and Kent R. Olson, MD

Intoxication by many different drugs and poisons may cause nausea or vomiting.[1-4] A variety of mechanisms may be involved: corrosive or irritant injury to the stomach; injury to the intestines, liver, pancreas, or other organs; mechanical obstruction; or central nervous system or generalized intoxication. Frequently, gastrointestinal disturbance plays only a minor role in the poisoning syndrome, but it provides an important clue to the diagnosis. In other cases, toxin-induced gastroenteritis may be profound and result in serious complications or death.

This chapter provides an overview of the common mechanisms of toxin-induced nausea and vomiting. Tables illustrate the variety of substances involved. The text highlights some of the most common specific substances and provides an approach to diagnosis and treatment. In most cases, toxin-induced nausea and vomiting are effectively managed with intravenous fluid replacement and administration of common parenteral antiemetics. Occasionally, a specific antidote is available.

Corrosive or Irritant Injury to Esophagus or Stomach

A large number of drugs, plants, mushrooms, minerals, and commercial and industrial products have corrosive or irritating effects on the gastrointestinal tract (Table 1).[5,6]

Ingestion of a strong acid, alkali, or other highly corrosive material typically causes severe pain in the throat, chest, and stomach. Crystalline solid products cause primarily throat and esophageal damage, whereas liquid products are also likely to injure the stomach and upper small intestine. If perforation of the esophagus or stomach occurs, the victim may develop hematemesis, tachycardia, shock, pancreatitis, or signs of peritonitis. Immediate surgery and extensive repair may be necessary. If the patient is stable but has persistent pain, endoscopy should be performed to determine the extent of damage. Deep or circumferential burns of the

Table 1. Corrosive or Irritant Agents

Category	Examples	Comments
Acids	Hydrochloric acid, sulfuric acid	Coagulative type eschar; may cause acidemia.
	Hydrofluoric acid	Delayed onset, progressive; may cause systemic hypocalcemia, hyperkalemia.
Alcohols	Ethanol, ethylene glycol, isopropyl alcohol, methanol	Ethylene glycol and methanol cause severe metabolic acidosis.
Alkalis	Sodium hydroxide, ammonia	Penetrating liquefactive necrosis.
Antiseptics/ disinfectants	Hydrogen peroxide, iodine, phenol, formaldehyde	Ingestion of hydrogen peroxide can cause gastricrupture due to liberation of oxygen. Phenol may produce seizures.
Borates	Borax, boric acid, polyborate	Lobster-red skin coloration, diarrhea, renal failure.
Dipyridil herbicides	Paraquat, diquat	Paraquat may cause progressive, fatal lung fibrosis. Diquat is associated with brain infarction, renal failure.
Essential oils/lubricants	Camphor, pennyroyal oil, wintergreen	Camphor can cause seizures. Pennyroyal oil is hepatotoxic. Wintergreen contains salicylate.
Hydrocarbons	Gasoline, kerosene, lighter fluid, furniture polish	Burping and irritation are common. Pulmonary aspiration can cause severe chemical pneumonia.

esophagus are likely to cause permanent scarring and resulting partial obstruction.[5,6] Treatment of ingestion of corrosive products consists of rapid dilution with plain water, followed by gastric lavage to remove residual stomach contents. There is no proven role for steroids in preventing stricture formation.[7]

Many corrosive products also produce serious systemic toxicity. For example, absorption of ingested phenol can cause seizures, coma, and cardiac disturbances. Paraquat causes progressive and irreversible lung fibrosis. Oxidizing agents can cause hemolysis and methemoglobinemia.[4]

Alcohols do not produce a highly corrosive injury but frequently cause gastric irritation.[8] Gastritis with hematemesis is most commonly described after ingestion of isopropyl alcohol.[9] The "toxic" alcohols methanol and ethylene glycol are metabolized to dangerous products such as formate and

Table 1. *Continued*

Category	Examples	Comments
Metals	Iron, lead, mercury, copper, arsenic, thallium, cadmium	Iron and lead are often visible on x-ray films. Copper salts often produce blue vomitus.
Mothballs	Naphthalene, paradichloroben-zene	Naphthalene may cause hemolysis in persons with low tolerance for oxidant stress.
Mushrooms	Numerous species	Most symptoms occur rapidly; delayed onset of vomiting (more than 8–12 hours) suggests *Amanita Phalloides*-type poisoning.
Nonsteroidal antiflamma-tory agents	Ibuprofen, naproxen, mefenamic acid	Massive overdose may cause acidosis, renal failure. Mefenamic acid may cause seizures.
Oxidizing agents	Bromates, chlorates, potassium permanganate	May also cause hemolysis, methemoglobinemia.
Plants	Daffodil bulbs, holly berries, mistletoe, pokeweed, hemlock, castor beans	Vomiting is usually accompanied by severe diarrhea. Hemlock may cause seizures, muscle spasms.
Pyrethrin insecticides	Derivatives of chrysanthemum	
Salicylates	Aspirin, wintergreen oil	Associated with metabolic acidosis, hyperpyrexia, pulmonary edema.

oxalate, which cause severe, multisystem organ damage. The diagnosis of such alcohol poisoning is suggested by the presence of elevated serum osmolality and a large anion gap metabolic acidosis.[3] Treatment of methanol or ethylene glycol poisoning includes administration of ethanol (to block metabolism of the parent compounds) and hemodialysis (to remove the parent compounds and their toxic products).

Ingested metal salts frequently cause irritant or corrosive gastrointestinal injury. Besides causing serious loss of blood and fluid volume due to corrosive gastroenteritis, these chemicals are often highly toxic when absorbed. For example, when mercuric chloride, which is used in stool collection jars as a fixative, is mistakenly ingested, severe, acute abdominal pain and vomiting occur. Absorption of the toxic mercuric salt causes acute proteinuria, hematuria, and oliguric renal failure. Diagnosis of systemic metal intoxication is based on the history of exposure and the presence of excess concentrations of metal compounds in the urine or blood. After acute ingestion, many of these compounds frequently may be visible on plain abdominal radiographs. Treatment consists of aggressive replacement of lost fluids, as well as specific chelating agents such as deferoxamine (for iron), dimercaprol (for lead, mercury, or arsenic), ethylenediamine tetra-acetic acid (EDTA) (for lead or mercury), or dimercaptosuccinic acid (DMSA) (for lead, mercury, or arsenic).[10]

Many species of plants and mushrooms cause gastroenteritis. Symptoms may be due to irritating chemicals or oils on the plant surface or contained in the leaves or stems. Ingestion of plants containing calcium oxalate crystals, such as dieffenbachia, may cause painful swelling in the mouth and throat. Poison oak and poison ivy contain resins that induce an inflammatory reaction in sensitized individuals. Castor beans contain the cathartic castor oil as well as the highly toxic substance ricin, both of which can cause severe abdominal cramps, vomiting, and diarrhea. Plant products or herbal medications may contain various essential oils, such as camphor or pennyroyal oil, that have systemic effects as well as local irritant actions. Treatment of plant-induced gastroenteritis is generally supportive, with aggressive fluid replacement and correction of electrolyte abnormalities.[4] In cases of methyl salicylate (oil of wintergreen) exposure, treatment is as for salicylates.

Consumption of salicylates and other nonsteroidal anti-inflammatory agents can cause gastritis and ulceration. Excessive salicylate use or acute overdose can produce severe anion gap metabolic acidosis, coma, seizures, hyperpyrexia, pulmonary edema, and death.[11] The serum salicylate concentration should be obtained immediately if salicylate poisoning is suspected. Treatment consists of alkalinization of the serum and urine to prevent salicylate from entering the brain and to enhance renal elimination. If the serum concentration is greater than 1000 mg/L (100 mg/dL) after an acute overdose or greater than 600 mg/L (60 mg/dL) with chronic accidental over medication, hemodialysis may be indicated.

Other Organ Damage

Besides causing simple irritation or corrosive injury to the esophagus or stomach, poisons may induce acute nausea or vomiting because of injury to other gastrointestinal organs or organ systems (Table 2).

Mesenteric intestinal ischemia can be caused by ergot derivatives, sympathomimetic agents, digitalis glycosides, or drugs that induce profound or prolonged hypotension. Patients with ergot-induced intestinal ischemia are often using excessive doses of ergot-containing products for treatment of

Table 2. Organ System Damage

Category	Examples	Comments
Intestinal ischemia	Ergotism	Most commonly seen with chronic excessive use or abuse of combination products containing barbiturates.
	Amphetamines, cocaine	Sympathomimetic overdose is usually accompanied by hypertension, tachycardia, agitation.
	Digitalis glycosides	Occasionally seen in patients on chronic therapy.
Inhibition of intestinal cell protein synthesis	Radioactive compounds	May occur after massive external irradiation or ingestion of radioactive isotopes.
	Colchicine	Severe diarrhea may occur after only a few milligrams.
	Antineoplastic agents	
	Amanita phalloides-type mushrooms	Massive gastroenteritis; amatoxin also causes massive hepatic necrosis.
Hepatic necrosis	Acetaminophen	Toxic single dose of 7–8 gm or 150 mg/kg; may also cause renal failure.
	Amanita phalloides-type mushrooms	Severe hepatic necrosis, often requiring liver transplantation.
	CCl_4, other chlorinated hydrocarbons	
Kidney failure	Amphetamines, cocaine, phencyclidine	Rhabdomyolysis with myoglobinuria, or hyperpyrexia-induced kidney damage.
	Arsine, stibine gases	Acute massive hemolysis with hemoglobinuria.
Pancreatitis	Numerous drugs and poisons with direct or metabolically activated toxicity: alcohols, salicylates, acetaminophen, scorpion stings, etc.	May occur with acute overdose or after chronic therapeutic use.
	Strong acids or alkalis	Penetrating corrosive injury with posterior gastric perforation.
Aortic rupture	Amphetamines, cocaine	Hypertensive acute dissection.
	Strong acids or alkalis	Penetrating corrosive injury.
Myocardial ischemia or infarction	Amphetamines, cocaine	Diffuse subendocardial injury or localized transmural infarction.

migraine. Another possibility is intentional abuse of the barbiturate butal-bital in the combination product Cafergot. Signs of ergotism include cold and pale extremities. Amphetamine or cocaine-induced bowel ischemia is typically accompanied by other signs of sympathomimetic intoxication, such as hypertension, tachycardia, sweating, and agitation. In most cases, symptoms improve after the offending drug is discontinued, but bowel resection has been required when severe ischemia resulted in bowel necrosis and gangrene.[2]

Substances that may interfere with protein synthesis, and block normal replacement of intestinal cell turnover, include alpha and beta particle-emitting radioactive isotopes, gamma rays, mitotic inhibitors such as colchicine, protein synthesis inhibitors such as *Amanita phalloides* mushroom, and many antineoplastic agents. In cases of toxicity, after a delay of several hours victims develop massive gastroenteritis, caused by sloughing of intestinal cells and loss of gut wall integrity. In addition to vomiting, there is voluminous diarrhea, which is often described as cholera-like or similar in appearance to thin rice-water. Treatment consists of aggressive intravenous fluid replacement, as well as specific management of other complications (such as leukopenia with radiation injury or hepatic necrosis with *Amanita phalloides* mushrooms).

Hepatic necrosis may be caused by a wide variety of drugs and chemical agents. Injury may be caused by direct cellular toxicity or by the generation of a toxic intermediate during metabolism of the parent compound. Acetaminophen, for example, is converted into a highly reactive intermediate during microsomal metabolism. Normally, the toxic intermediate is scavenged by intracellular glutathione and excreted as a nontoxic mercapturic compound. With overdose, however, glutathione stores are depleted, and the intermediate then attacks liver cells. Signs of hepatotoxicity are often delayed for 2 to 3 days; initial symptoms after acute acetaminophen overdose may be absent or consist only of nausea and vomiting. If acetaminophen ingestion is suspected, the serum acetaminophen concentration should be obtained immediately. If the acetaminophen level 4 hours after ingestion is greater than 150 mg/L, treatment with the antidote n-acetylcysteine is indicated.[12] N-acetylcysteine, which acts as a substitute scavenger of the toxic metabolite, should be given within 8 to 10 hours of ingestion to be most effective.

Ingestion of even part of a cap of *Amanita phalloides* or other amatoxin-containing mushrooms can lead to massive hepatic necrosis, hepatic encephalopathy, and death. There is no effective antidote for the amatoxin poison, which inhibits cellular protein synthesis by specific action on RNA. Orthotopic liver transplantation has been lifesaving in several cases.

Manifestations of acute renal failure may include abdominal and flank pain, nausea, and vomiting. The most common poison-related causes of acute renal failure are ingestion of mercuric salts, rhabdomyolysis from sympathomimetic overdose, and massive hemolysis from exposure to oxidizing agents or to the highly toxic gases arsine (arsenic hydride) or stibine (antimony hydride). Treatment of rhabdomyolysis includes administration of large volumes of fluids to maintain a high urine flow and alkalinization of the urine to prevent deposition of the toxic myoglobin in the tubules. Acute hemoglobinuria and flank pain are common in patients with massive hemolysis, as are nausea and vomiting. Treatment of hemoglobinuria is similar to that for rhabdomyolysis. In addition, blood transfusions may be needed if the hematocrit falls below 25 g/dL. Chelating agents such as those used for arsenic poisoning (e.g., dimercaprol) are not effective.[4]

Pancreatitis is a complication of numerous drugs taken therapeutically or in overdose. The mechanisms are diverse. Some drugs, such as the alcohols, are directly toxic to the pancreas, and toxicity usually occurs promptly after exposure and is dose related.[13] Other cases may be due to generation of a toxic metabolite or may be idiosyncratic or hypersensitivity reactions. The presentation may be either sudden or chronic and subacute. Most patients have abdominal epigastric pain, nausea and vomiting, and elevated serum amylase concentrations. Drugs associated with pancreatitis include acetaminophen, azothioprine, cimetidine, corticosteroids, procainamide, salicylates, and tetracycline.[14] Scorpion stings also can cause pancreatitis.

Cardiovascular system disturbances can also cause nausea and vomiting. Sympathomimetic-induced myocardial ischemia or infarction or aortic and other large vessel dissection can result in acute chest or abdominal pain accompanied by diaphoresis, nausea, and vomiting. Frequently, the onset of cocaine-induced myocardial ischemia is delayed until several hours after the initial exposure, when other signs of acute sympathomimetic intoxication may be absent or waning. Electrocardiographic evidence may be nonspecific, especially with diffuse myocardial necrosis or subendocardial injury.

Mechanical Obstruction

Mechanical gastrointestinal tract obstruction should be suspected in any patient presenting with unexplained nausea and vomiting, especially children. While ingestion of foreign objects such as coins is usually benign, small objects can cause significant medical problems. An example is lead fishing or curtain weights, which can be retained in the stomach long enough for the lead to be oxidized by stomach acid and absorbed systemically. Fatal encephalopathy from swallowing of a lead curtain weight has been reported.[15] In most instances, conservative treatment-bulk laxatives to encourage passage, serial x-ray studies to monitor progress, and measurement of lead levels in the blood to assess absorption is sufficient until the weight is passed in the stool. However, more aggressive measures, such as endoscopic or surgical removal, may be indicated for prolonged retention of the weight in the stomach or for elevated lead levels.

Disc batteries are another commonly swallowed foreign body.[16] In the vast majority of patients, the batteries pass through the gastrointestinal tract without problems. However, the larger diameter batteries (>15 mm) can lodge in the esophagus, where they can open up and leak corrosive contents. Fatalities have occurred due to perforation and exsanguination. Once the batteries pass beyond the esophagus, serious problems are unlikely. An initial x-ray film should be done to determine the location of the battery. Batteries located in the esophagus should be removed immediately via esophagoscopy; the course of other batteries may be monitored with x-ray studies to document passage. Although many batteries contain heavy metals such as mercury, there have been no reported cases of systemic metal poisoning.

Radiographs can also help diagnose mechanical obstruction in "body packers" or "mules," who swallow drug-filled condoms or packets for smuggling.[17] In addition to life-threatening systemic toxicity from rupture of the containers and release of their contents, these balloons have caused mechanical gastrointestinal obstruction. Treatment of asymptomatic patients involves administration of activated charcoal with sorbitol or other cathartics or whole bowel irrigation, until the passage of all bags is verified on x-ray studies. Individuals with serious symptoms of intoxication or mechanical obstruction may require surgical intervention.

Certain drugs tend to clump together to form bezoars, especially when taken in overdoses. These concretions not only complicate the management of the overdose by delaying or prolonging systemic toxicity, but they can also result in intestinal obstruction.[18] Aspirin, iron, and aluminum hydroxide are often implicated as causing drug bezoars. Diagnosis of drug bezoars can be made by plain abdominal radiography in some instances, but contrast studies may be required.[19]

Drugs with strong anticholinergic characteristics, including tricyclic antidepressants and phenothiazine antipsychotics, are frequently associated with constipation during therapeutic usage. In severe cases, adynamic ileus and intestinal obstruction can ensue. A case of thioridazine-induced abdominal distention resulting in aortic obstruction has been reported.[2]

Activated charcoal is used as a method of gastrointestinal decontamination after ingestion of a variety of toxins, and repetitive-dose treatment has been advocated to increase the clearance of some drugs after overdoses. Though inherently benign, overly zealous use of activated charcoal can result in gastrointestinal obstruction. The risk is especially high for those drugs with anticholinergic properties, such as carbamazepine and amitriptyline. Because repetitive doses of activated charcoal have not been shown to alter clinical outcome in most cases of overdose, the benefits of this treatment should be carefully weighed against the risks of mechanical obstruction and other complications.[20]

Systemic Intoxication

A wide variety of pharmaceutical, chemical, and biological agents can cause nausea and vomiting as manifestations of systemic toxicity (Table 3).

Drugs

Acetaminophen overdose is an exceedingly common problem. Other than nausea and vomiting, there are no specific symptoms or clinical findings early after ingestion. As a result, the diagnosis is frequently missed, and treatment with the antidote N-acetylcysteine is often delayed, increasing the likelihood of hepatic damage. Severe and persistent nausea and vomiting can seriously interfere with the oral administration of the antidote. Slow administration of the antidote via nasogastric tube, along with a parenteral antiemetic such as metoclopramide, is usually effective. Occasionally, N-acetylcysteine has to be given by intravenous infusion.

Digoxin and, less commonly, digitoxin are used for treatment of congestive heart failure and atrial arrhythmias. A number of plants contain cardiac glycosides with actions similar to that of digoxin: examples include foxglove, oleander, rhododendron, and azalea. Poisoning in humans from ingestion of plant material is uncommon, unless the plants are deliberately eaten or the toxins are concentrated, for example, by the making of tea. In acute overdose, sinus and atrioventricular block and potentially life-threatening hyperkalemia are more likely to be seen than are ventricular dysrhythmias. In chronic overdose, which usually occurs in patients with underlying heart disease, ventricular tachyarrhythmias are more common, and they often are seen at digoxin blood levels much lower than those in acute overdose. Digibind (fragments of digoxin-specific antibodies) is indicated for severe toxicity unresponsive to standard therapy.[21] It may also reverse the toxic effects of other glycosides found in cardiotoxic plants.

Syrup of ipecac, while recognized as a generally safe and effective drug for inducing emesis, has infrequently resulted in Mallory-Weiss tear or

Table 3. Systemic Intoxication

Intoxicant	Comments
Drugs	
Acetaminophen	Nausea and vomiting may be the only early symptoms. Liver injury is apparent after 2–3 days.
Calcium channel antagonists	Hypotension and bradycardia are primary findings. Nausea, vomiting, mental status changes, metabolic acidosis also occur.
Digoxin and digitoxin	Acute and chronic overdoses present differently. Nausea and vomiting are very common with both. Acute: supraventricular arrhythmias, heart block, bradycardia, hyperkalemia. Chronic: all types of arrhythmias, weakness, visual disturbances.
Ethanol-disulfiram	Rapid onset of vomiting, flushing, hypotension from accumulation of acetaldehyde. Rarely, can lead to myocardial infarction or arrhythmias.
Fluoride	Ingestion of more than 5 mg/kg can cause profuse vomiting, shock, hypocalcemia.
Ipecac	Abused by anorexics/bulimics, implicated in child abuse (Munchausen-by-proxy syndrome). Long-term abuse can result in cardiomyopathy, arrhythmias.
Methemoglobinemia inducers	Examples: phenazopyridine, dapsone, benzocaine. Signs and symptoms of hypoxia worsen as methemoglobin concentration rises. Treatment with methylene blue normally is not needed unless the concentration is over 30%.
Opioid drug withdrawal	Intense abdominal cramps, nausea, vomiting, piloerection, agitation and insomnia are common.
Phenytoin	Nausea, vomiting, nystagmus, and ataxia are common.
Quinidine and other type 1A antiarrhythmias	Gastrointestinal disturbances are very common with acute or chronic overdose. Severe toxicity is associated with wide QRS and QT intervals and hypotension, atrioventricular block, ventricular arrhythmias.
Theophylline and caffeine	Nausea and vomiting are very common, especially after acute overdose. Seizures and arrhythmias can occur with very high levels.
Thyroid	T^3 (liothyronine) overdose, results in toxicity within the first 6 hours. Intoxication with T^4 (levothyroxine), which is converted to T^3, can be delayed 1–3 days. Tachycardia or hyperthermia may occur.

Table 3. *Continued*

Intoxicant	Comments
Chemicals	
Arsenic	Nausea and vomiting are common in both acute and chronic intoxications. In acute overdose, profound fluid and electrolyte loss may quickly result in death. Multiorgan disturbances, most profoundly peripheral sensory neuropathy, are common.
Carbon monoxide	Early symptoms include nausea, vomiting, headache, dizziness; can progress to coma, seizures, arrhythmias. Neuropsychiatric sequelae can result.
Cyanide	Abrupt onset of symptoms soon after exposure. Symptoms include nausea, dyspnea, confusion, coma, seizures, cardiopulmonary arrest.
Hydrogen sulfide	Mechanism of action and toxicity similar to those of cyanide.
Lead	Gastrointestinal disturbances are common with acute and chronic exposures. Colic and constipation, along with anemia and peripheral neuropathy, are seen with chronic exposure.
Metal fumes	Acute febrile illness with nausea, vomiting, and chills, results from inhalation of metal oxides. Most commonly seen with inhalation of zinc oxide while welding, this is generally a self-limited disease.
Pesticides	Organophosphates/carbamates: Rapid onset of gastrointestinal disturbances, excessive fluid production, central nervous system depression, seizures, respiratory arrest can occur.
	Organochlorines (lindane, chlordane): Vomiting is very common with ingestion. Altered mental status, and seizures are common. Cardiac dysrhythmias from myocardial sensitivity to catecholamines may be seen.
	Metaldehyde: Widely available as snail baits, this pesticide when ingested may cause metabolic acidosis and seizures.
	Methyl bromide, ethylene dibromide (fumigants): Malaise, nausea, vomiting, headache, tremor, seizures, coma, and pulmonary edema are possible consequences of exposure.
	Nicotine: An extremely potent insecticide, it is rapidly absorbed orally and dermally. Rapid onset of symptoms occurs from initial excitation then depression of nicotinic cholinergic receptors.

Table 3. *Continued*

Intoxicant	Comments
Solvents	Toluene/xylene: These are commonly used solvents in household products. Toluene is also abused for its euphoric potential. Ataxia, coma, respiratory arrest, myocardial sensitization can occur.
	Trichloroethane: Used in dry cleaning and also in many household items like upholstery protectors. This chemical has high potential for abuse. Sudden death from myocardial sensitization has been seen.
Sodium azide	This chemical is used in automobile air bags and also as a preservative. Persistent nausea and vomiting may be the only symptoms before death from acute cardiomyopathy.
Biologicals **Bites and Stings**	
Black widow spider	Progressively painful muscle cramping and fasciculations occur within 1–2 hours of a bite. Nausea, vomiting, board-like rigidity of abdomen and back, and hypertension are seen.
Jellyfish	Immediate burning pain can be followed by nausea, vomiting, paresthesias, hypotension, muscle spasm. Death is rare except with box jellyfish.
Scorpion	Most stings result in local pain only. Stings from *Centuroides* sp. (southwestern US and Mexico) can cause more severe systemic symptoms, including vomiting, agitation, hypersalivation.
Snake	Nausea, vomiting, and metallic taste, in addition to local pain, are initial symptoms of venomous snake bites. Can progress to tissue necrosis, coagulopathy, shock.
Food Poisoning	
Bacteria	Staphylococcus aureus and bacillus cereus bacteria produced preformed toxins in food, resulting in rapid onset of nausea and vomiting.
Mushrooms	*Amanita phalloides* and related sp, *Galerina autumnalis, Lepiota,* sp; contain amatoxin. Profound vomiting, diarrhea, abdominal symptoms are hallmarks. Hepatic failure ensues.
	Clitocybe, Inocybe sp: Contain muscarine. Muscarinic symptoms along with vomiting and diarrhea.

Table 3. *Continued*

Intoxicants	Comments
	Amanita muscaria: Contains anticholinergic alkaloids. Cause hallucinations, dilated pupils, flushed dry skin, tachycardia. Vomiting is common early after ingestion.
	Gyrometra sp: Contain hepatotoxic mono-methylhydrazine.
	Coprinus sp ("inky cap"): Produce disulfiram-like reaction when ingested with alcohol.
Seafood	Ciguatera: Results from ingestion of reef fish, mostly in tropical areas. Vomiting and watery diarrhea 1–6 hours after ingestion is followed by malaise, myalgias, paresthesias, autonomic dysfunction, and reversal of hot and cold sensations.
	Domoic acid: Ingestion of shellfish contaminated with toxin-producing dinoflagellates. Nausea, vomiting, and diarrhea, followed by paralysis, seizures and permanent memory loss, have occurred.
	Paralytic shellfish: Ingestion of bivalve mollusks contaminated with saxitoxin. Vomiting, diarrhea, and facial paresthesia occur within 30 minutes of ingestion. Respiratory paralysis can occur in serious cases.
	Scombroid: Results when fish tissue decomposes, producing histamine and histamine-like compounds. Vomiting, flushing, and hypotension can result.
Plants	
Cardiac glycosides	Foxglove, oleander, rhododendron: Contain digoxin-like substances.
Nicotine-like	Poison hemlock, wild tobacco: Rapid onset of vomiting, central nervous system excitation, seizures, respiratory arrest can occur.
Cyanogenic glycosides	*Prunus* sp (almond, apricot, cherry, peach, apple), elderberry, hydrangea: These glycosides yield hydrocyanic acid upon hydrolysis. Toxicity as described above for cyanide.
Ipecacuanha	Syrup is widely used to induce vomiting. Excessive repeated use can cause cardiomyopathy, arrhythmias.

hemorrhagic gastritis with therapeutic use. In addition, persistent nausea and emesis from ipecac may interfere with subsequent administration of activated charcoal. Chronic repeated use of ipecac syrup by bulimic patients has resulted in accumulation of cardiotoxic alkaloids and fatal cardiomyopathy and arrhythmias. Intentional poisoning of children with ipecac has been reported and should be considered in children with unexplained chronic vomiting and diarrhea.[22]

Quinidine, procainamide, and disopyramide are type 1A antiarrhythmic agents, all of which have low toxic therapeutic ratios. Severe and often fatal intoxication can occur at doses only slightly above therapeutic levels. Even at therapeutic doses, these drugs frequently cause gastroenteritis, which may necessitate cessation of therapy. With acute overdose, nausea, vomiting, and diarrhea are very common. By slowing sodium-dependent phase 0 depolarization and subsequent repolarization of the cardiac action potential, these drugs can significantly inhibit conduction velocity and contractility, resulting in hypotension and cardiac arrhythmias. Rapid gut decontamination and intensive supportive care are essential in cases of overdose. Administration of hypertonic sodium bicarbonate may help overcome the effects of sodium channel blockade.

Theophylline overdose can present a significant challenge to the clinician. Acute overdoses result in nausea, vomiting, tachycardia, metabolic acidosis, hypokalemia, and hypotension. With theophylline levels above 100 mg/L, intractable seizures and ventricular arrhythmias are common. Chronic intoxication may occur as a result of excessive misuse by patients. Another cause of chronic theophylline intoxication is a decrease in normal hepatic metabolism, which may result from concomitant use of erythromycin or cimetidine, an acute viral infection, or hepatic insufficiency. Seizures can occur unpredictably in these patients, sometimes at serum theophylline levels only a little above or even within the therapeutic range. For those patients with severe toxicity, rapid removal of the drug by charcoal hemoperfusion or hemodialysis is indicated. Administration of multiple dose activated charcoal also hastens the elimination of theophylline, but the effectiveness of this procedure is not as rapid as with dialysis, and it can be difficult in the patient with protracted vomiting. Theophylline-induced vomiting has been successfully managed with parenteral ranitidine, an H^2 receptor blocker.[23]

Chemicals

Certain metals and metalloids, most notably lead, mercury, and arsenic, can cause serious illness. Arsenic-containing compounds may occur as pentavalent (arsenate) or trivalent (arsenite) forms; the trivalent compounds are much more toxic than the pentavalent ones. Abrupt onset of nausea, vomiting, and watery diarrhea is characteristic of acute arsenic toxicity.[24] Chronic arsenic poisoning should be suspected in patients with a glove or stocking pattern of peripheral sensory neuropathy, weakness, anorexia, nausea, vomiting, and alopecia. Neurologic damage may persist despite treatment with chelating agents.

Lead poisoning is a more widespread problem due to the ubiquitous presence of this metal.[25] Chronic lead intoxication can cause nausea, abdominal colic, anemia (microcytic or normocytic), and peripheral motor neuropathy. As a result of recent studies linking low-level lead exposure in children to their impaired intellectual development, the Centers for Disease Control have lowered the definition of an "acceptable" blood lead concentration to 10 mcg/dL; at this level, no symptoms are discernible. Treatment of lead intoxication may require chelation with calcium disodium EDTA, dimercaprol, or dimercaptosuccinic acid.

Poisoning by gases such as carbon monoxide, cyanide, or hydrogen sulfide needs to be recognized and treated quickly if permanent injury or death is to be averted. Each of these gases produces cellular asphyxia. At low levels of exposure, most persons experience headache, nausea, vomiting, dyspnea, and confusion. At higher levels, syncope, coma, and seizures may occur. Carbon monoxide is produced by combustion of any organic material, and so poisoning should be suspected in victims of smoke inhalation or whenever a motor is running in an enclosed area. Administration of 100% oxygen via a tight-fitting non-rebreather mask or by endotracheal tube will rapidly reduce the half-life of carboxyhemoglobin. The use of a hyperbaric oxygen chamber to deliver higher oxygen concentrations remains controversial.

Cyanide is also produced in fires and is an important toxin in smoke inhalation victims. Cyanide salts are used in chemical laboratories, metal plating, and a variety of other industrial situations. Acetonitrile, a component in artificial nail removers, is converted to cyanide after ingestion. Many plants contain cyanogenic glycosides (see Table 3). Treatment of cyanide intoxication includes administration of oxygen and the antidotes amyl or sodium nitrite (which create methemoglobin, which binds free cyanide) and sodium thiosulfate (which promotes conversion of cyanide to less toxic thiocyanate).[4]

Many insecticides are capable of producing profound toxicity in humans.[26] Organophosphates irreversibly bind acetylcholinesterase, and carbamates bind to it reversibly. Therefore, initial signs and symptoms of toxicity caused by these insecticide compounds are indistinguishable, although the duration of toxicity may differ. By binding to acetylcholinesterase, these insecticides cause excessive accumulation of acetylcholine at muscarinic and nicotinic receptors and in the central nervous system. Muscarinic (parasympathetic) manifestations include salivation, lacrimation, urination, and diarrhea (a syndrome abbreviated SLUD), along with vomiting, abdominal cramping, miosis, bradycardia, bronchorrhea, and bronchospasm. Nicotinic (ganglionic) effects include muscle fasciculation, tachycardia, and respiratory muscle paralysis, the usual cause of death. Among central nervous system effects are ataxia, seizures, and coma. Atropine, often in extremely large doses, is used to reverse the muscarinic effects. Antidotal treatment for organophosphates involves pralidoxime, which enables regeneration of acetylcholinesterase.

Organochlorines, or chlorinated hydrocarbon insecticides, represent some of the most toxic and ecologically damaging insecticides. Some, including DDT and chlordane, are now banned from commercial use due to their persistence in and damage to the environment. Lindane, however, is still commonly used for the treatment of lice and scabies. Ingestion of as little as 100 mg, or 10 mL of the 1% lotion or shampoo, is potentially epileptogenic in a child.[27] Chlorinated hydrocarbons cause vomiting when ingested, and may also cause arrhythmias and hepatic damage. Because no specific antidotes are available, rapid decontamination of the gut with gastric lavage is essential; induction of emesis is contraindicated due to the potential for abrupt onset of seizures. Activated charcoal or cholestyramine may interrupt enterohepatic recirculation and enhance elimination.

Metaldehyde, which is used as a snail and slug killer, commonly causes protracted vomiting. It can also produce seizures and metabolic acidosis.

Rarely used now as a pesticide, nicotine is an exceedingly toxic substance. Ingestion of as little as 2 to 5 mg of concentrated liquid nicotine can cause symptoms. Intoxication has occurred in children from ingestion of cigarettes and in farm workers who were harvesting tobacco. The literature describes illness in a person who sat on a chair where a nicotine solution had been spilled.[28] Nicotine initially stimulates the sympathetic nervous system, then the parasympathetic. Ganglionic and neuromuscular blockade results with higher doses. Direct effects on the brain can cause vomiting and seizures. Abdominal cramps, vomiting, diarrhea, diaphoresis, and salivation are common with small doses. With severe poisoning, seizures, coma, cardiovascular collapse, and respiratory muscle paralysis can lead to death. No specific antidote is available.

Aliphatic, aromatic, and chlorinated hydrocarbons are used as solvents in a large number of commercial products, including oil-based paints, insecticides, typewriter correction fluid, upholstery protectant, and adhesives. Patients who believe they have been poisoned by inhaling the vapors of insecticides often exhibit symptoms more closely related to exposure to solvents. These symptoms include nausea, euphoria, dizziness, and head-ache. Treatment consists simply of removal from the source. Excessive inhalation of solvent vapors in enclosed, unventilated spaces or deliberate insufflation to create euphoria can result in coma and cardiac arrhythmias.

Bites and Stings

Nausea and vomiting are frequent manifestations of a variety of envenom-ations. Black widow and brown recluse spiders are the two most significant species of venomous spiders in the United States. Black widow bites result in no initial pain but rapid onset of muscle cramping and fasciculations. When the cramping progresses toward the chest, back, or abdomen, the symptoms can mimic myocardial infarction or an acute abdominal condi-tion. Treatment consists of pain relievers, skeletal muscle relaxants and, at times, antihypertensive agents.[29] Although available, black widow antive-nin is rarely used. Brown recluse bites can result in a progressive, severely necrotic ulcer at the bite site and systemic symptoms such as nausea, vomiting, and dizziness. Rarely, generalized rash, fever, lymphadenopathy, jaundice, and hemolysis may follow.

Rattlesnakes and other pit vipers (Crotalidae) are the most common indigenous poisonous snakes in the United States. Although nausea and vomiting are relatively common symptoms of envenomation, they are usu-ally overshadowed by local pain, swelling, and ecchymosis. Other systemic manifestations of rattlesnake envenomation include perioral tingling, muscle fasciculations, weakness, and coagulopathy. Polyvalent Crotalidae antivenin can reverse all the symptoms, although concerns about serum sickness and, rarely, anaphylaxis limit its universal acceptance.[30]

Jellyfish and other Cnidaria, including fire coral, Portuguese man-of-war, and anemones are capable of inflicting painful stings with venom that is contained in microscopic structures called nematocysts. The nematocysts are contained within outer sacs arranged along the tentacles or the surface of these animals. When they are disturbed, the nematocysts release venom. Immediate stinging and burning pain can be followed by paresthesia, hy-potension, muscle spasms, nausea, vomiting, abdominal pain, myalgia, and, rarely, coma, seizures, and arrhythmias. The degree of the illness is determined by the number of nematocysts involved.[4]

Food Poisoning

Of an estimated 5,000 species of mushrooms found in the United States, about 100 are potentially toxic. The majority of toxic mushrooms cause

mild to moderate self-limited gastroenteritis within a few hours of ingestion. However, a few species may cause severe or fatal poisoning. As discussed earlier, mushrooms containing amatoxin, including many *Amanita*
and *Galerina* species, are highly toxic. Characteristically, onset of severe
vomiting, abdominal cramps, and diarrhea is delayed at least 8 to 12 hours
after ingestion. A victim who survives the intense gastroenteritis may develop fulminant hepatic necrosis. Another type of mushroom, *Gyrometra
esculenta,* contains monomethylhydrazine, which may also cause delayed-
onset gastroenteritis. Subsequent development of weakness, seizures, hemolysis, and methemoglobinemia can ensue.

Some genera of mushrooms (*clitocybe, inocybe*) contain muscarine,
which stimulates muscarinic cholinergic receptors, resulting in salivation,
sweating, abdominal cramps, vomiting, diarrhea, and miosis soon after
ingestion. Although atropine may alleviate the symptoms, specific treatment is rarely needed. The *Amanita muscaria* mushroom contains little
muscarine but instead produces an anticholinergic syndrome caused by
ibotenic acid and other alkaloids. It also contains emetic alkaloids, which
limit its widespread use as a hallucinogen. Interestingly, *Coprinus* species
elaborate coprine, which produces a disulfiram-like interaction when ingested with ethanol.[1]

A poisoning that was once localized to tropical areas but is now more
widespread is ciguatera fish poisoning. The ciguatera toxin is produced by
small organisms called dinoflagellates that are consumed by reef fish. After
eating contaminated fish, the victim experiences nausea, vomiting, and
watery diarrhea; this is typically followed by weakness, paresthesia, autonomic dysfunction, and severe pruritus. Although not truly pathogno-
monic, reversal of hot and cold sensation is highly suggestive of ciguatera
poisoning. These symptoms can last for weeks or, by some accounts, years.
Unfortunately, no specific antidotal therapy is available.[31]

A common though poorly recognized fish poisoning is scombroid.
Scombrotoxin is a mixture of histamine and histamine-like compounds
produced when histidine in fish tissue decomposes. Those fish with pink
or red flesh, such as tuna, are more likely to produce scombrotoxin. The
symptoms of poisoning are rapid onset of nausea, vomiting, prickly sensation of oral mucous membranes, flushing, and urticaria. Although the
symptoms generally subside after a few hours, treatment with histamine
antagonists such as cimetidine or diphenhydramine have been reported to
hasten recovery.

Shellfish are responsible for several types of poisonings. On the Pacific
coast, the most common of these is paralytic shellfish poisoning. During the
warmer months, dinoflagellates produce saxitoxin, which is concentrated

by filter-feeding bivalves like clams and mussels. Ingestion of the affected mollusks results in rapid onset of facial paresthesia, vomiting, and diarrhea. In severe cases, muscle weakness may result in respiratory arrest. Treatment is supportive. Recently, an outbreak of serious illness in Canada led to the identification of a new shellfish-carried poison named domoic acid. This poison is thought to be elaborated by dinoflagellates and concentrated by shellfish. Symptoms include nausea, vomiting, paralysis, seizures, and, rarely, death. Some of the victims suffered permanent memory loss. No specific treatment is available.[32]

References

1. Ellenhorn MJ, Barceloux DG, eds. *Medical Toxicology.* New York: Elsevier; 1988.
2. Mueller PD, Benowitz NL. Toxicologic causes of acute abdominal disorders. *Emerg Med Clinics of North America.* 1989;7(3):667–683.
3. Olson KR, Pentel PR, Kelley MT. Physical assessment and differential diagnosis of the poisoned patient. *Med Toxicol.* 1987;2:52–76.
4. Olson KR, ed. *Poisoning & Drug Overdose.* Norwalk, Conn: Appleton & Lange; 1990.
5. Howell JM. Alkaline ingestions. *Ann Emerg Med.* 1986;15:820–825.
6. Wasserman RL, Ginsburg CM. Caustic substance injuries. *J Pediatr.* 1985;107(2):169–174.
7. Anderson, KD, Rouse TM, Randolph JG. A controlled trial of corticosteroids in children with corrosive injury of the esophagus. *N Engl J Med.* 1990;323:637–640.
8. Duffens K, Marx JA. Alcoholic ketoacidosis—a review. *J Emerg Med.* 1987;5:399–406.
9. Rich J, Scheife RT, Katz N, et al. Isopropyl alcohol intoxication. *Arch Neurol.* 1990;47:322–324.
10. Proudfoot AT, Simpson D, Dyson EH. Management of acute iron poisoning. *Med Toxicol.* 1986;1(2):83–100.
11. McGuigan MA. A two-year review of salicylate deaths in Ontario. *Arch Intern Med.* 1987;147:510–512.
12. Smilkstein MJ, Knapp GL, Kulig KW, et al. Efficacy of oral N-acetylcysteine in the treatment of acetaminophen overdose. *N Engl J Med.* 1988;319:1557–1562.
13. Caldarola V, Hassett JM, Hall AH, et al. Hemorrhagic pancreatitis associated with acetaminophen overdose. *Am J Gastroenterol.* 1986;81:579–582.
14. Mallory A, Kern F. Drug-induced pancreatitis: a critical review. *Gastroenterology.* 1980;78:813–820.
15. Hugelmeyer CD, Moorhead JC, Horenblas L, et al. Fatal lead encephalopathy following foreign body ingestion: case report. *J Emerg Med.* 1988;6:397–400.
16. Litovitz TL. Battery ingestions: product accessibility and clinical course. *Pediatrics.* 1985;75:469–476.
17. McCarron MM, Wood JD. The cocaine "body packer" syndrome. *JAMA.* 1983;250 (11):1417–1420.
18. Cereda JM, Scott J, Quigley EM. Endoscopic removal of pharmacobezoar of slow release theophylline. *Br Med J.* 1986;293:1143.
19. Korenman MD, Stubbs MB, Fish JC. Intestinal obstruction from medication bezoars. *JAMA.* 1978;240:54–55.
20. Watson WA, Cremer KF, Chapman JA. Gastrointestinal obstruction associated with multiple-dose activated charcoal. *J Emerg Med.* 1986;4:401–407.

21. Stolshek BS, Osterhout SK, Dunham G. The role of digoxin-specific antibodies in the treatment of digitalis poisoning. *Med Toxicol.* 1988;3:167–171.

22. Sutphen JL, Saulsbury FT. Intentional ipecac poisoning: Munchausen syndrome by proxy. *Pediatrics.* 1988;82(3pt 2):453–456.

23. Sessler CN. Theophylline toxicity: clinical features of 116 consecutive cases. *Am J Med.* 1990;88(6):567–576.

24. Campbell JP, Alvarez JA. Acute arsenic intoxication. *Am Fam Physician.* 1989;40(6):93–97.

25. Amitai Y, Graef JW, Brown MJ, et al. Hazards of "deleading" homes of children with lead poisoning. *Am J Dis Child.* 1987;141(7):758–760.

26. Mortensen ML. Management of acute childhood poisonings caused by selected insecticides and herbicides. *Pediatr Clin North Am.* 1986;33(2):421–445.

27. Sunder Ram Rao CV, Shreenivas R, Singh V, et al. Disseminated intravascular coagulation in a case of fatal lindane poisoning. *Vet Hum Toxicol.* 1988;30(2):132–134.

28. Ghosh SK, Parikh JR, Gokani VN, et al. Occupational health problems among tobacco processing workers: a preliminary study. *Arch Environ Health.* 1985;40(6):318–321.

29. Moss HS, Binder LS. A retrospective review of black widow spider envenomation. *Ann Intern Med.* 1987;16:188–192.

30. Wingert WA, Chan L. Rattlesnake bites in Southern California and rationale for recommended treatment. *West J Med.* 1988;148:37–44.

31. Hashimi MA, Sorokin JJ, Levin SM. Ciguatera fish poisoning. *N Engl J Med.* 1989;86(6):469–471.

32. Perl TM, Bedard L, Kosatsky T, et al. An outbreak of toxic encephalopathy caused by eating mussels contaminated with domoic acid. *N Engl J Med.* 1990;322(25):1775–1780.

Index

Abdomen, 1, 6
    distention of, 72
    motion sickness and muscles of, 44
    radiation-induced emesis and upper, 117
Abdominal colic, 153, 157
Abdominal cramps, 68, 146, 152, 154−160
Abdominal vagus nerve, 1, 2, 3, 8, 129
    See also Vagus nerve
Abortion, therapeutic, 95
Acetaldehyde, 152
Acetaminophen, 147, 151, 152, 156
    hepatic necrosis and, 148
    pancreatitis and, 149
Acetonuria, 77
Acetylcholine, 73, 130, 157−158
    metoclopramide and, 108
Achalasia, 64. *See also* Relaxation
Acid, 63
Acidemia, 144 (table)
Acidosis, metabolic, 144 (table), 145, 146, 152,
    153, 156
Acids (injury from), 144 (table), 147
ACTH. *See* Adrenocorticotropic hormone
    (ACTH)
Actinomycin-D, 127 (table)
Activated charcoal, 150−151, 156, 158
Acyclovir, 35
Adrenal activity, 52−53
Adrenergic blockage, 57
Adrenocorticotropic hormone (ACTH), 52, 53
Age
    and anticipatory nausea and vomiting, 17,
        18, 139
    chemotherapy-induced emesis and, 125
    and postoperative nausea and vomiting, 95
Agitation, 147, 148, 152, 154
Akathisia, 133
Alcohol, 19 (table), 125, 144 (table)
    poisoning from, 144−145, 147, 149, 152, 160
    pregnancy and, 87
Alkalis, 143, 144 (table), 147
Alkalosis, metabolic, 124
Alopecia, 157
Aluminum hydroxide, 150
Amatoxin, 147, 148, 154, 160
Amino acids, 80
Amitriptyline, 40, 151
Amphetamine, 38 (table), 58, 147
Ampullary nerve, 31
Amyloidosis, 67, 68
Analgesics, 38, 95 (table)
Androgens, 127 (table)
Anemia, 153, 157
Anesthesia, 96−99
    face mask in, 98

hypotension and, 104
    postoperative nausea and vomiting caused by,
        93, 94, 95
Angiography, 35, 36
Anorexia, 69, 124, 152, 157
Antacids, 95
Antiarrhythmias, type 1A, 152, 156
Anticholinergic agent, 38 (table), 65, 103, 130
    poisoning from, 150, 151, 154, 160
Anticipatory nausea and vomiting (ANV),
        11−23, 125, 139
    anxiety and, 16−17
    clinical characteristics of, 17−20
    conditioned by posttreatment emesis, 13−16,
        18, 20
    as learned response, 11, 12−17, 23
    lorazepam for, 133
    motion sickness and, 53
    treatment of, 20−23
Anticoagulation, 36
Antidepressant, 65, 72
Antiemetics, 33, 88
    after surgery, 105
    anesthesia for surgery and, 96, 99, 100
    chemotherapy-induced emesis and, 11, 20,
        123−140
    for migraine, 38, 39−40
    radiation-induced emesis and, 116, 117−118,
        120
    sympathomimetics as, 104
    See also specific ones
Antihistamines, 38 (table), 40, 160
Antihypertensive agent, 65
Antineoplastic drugs, 126, 147, 148
Antiplatelet therapy, 36
Antiseptics/disinfectants, 144 (table)
Antithyroid microsomal antibody, 79
Antivert, 38 (table)
Antivertigo drugs, 31, 38, 39−40
Antiviral agents, 35
ANV. *See* Anticipatory nausea and vomiting
    (ANV)
Anxiety
    anticipatory nausea and vomiting caused by,
        16−17, 21, 23
    gastrointestinal motility disorders and, 69
    lorazepam for, 133
    and postoperative nausea and vomiting,
        95 (table)
    and radiation-induced nausea and vomiting,
        113, 116
Aortic rupture, 147, 149
Apomorphine, 54
Appendicitis, 82
Appetite, 77

163

ephedrine and, 104
and postoperative nausea and vomiting, 94, 100, 101
radiation-induced emesis and, 115
treatment of, 56–59
Motoneurons, 7. *See also* Motor output
Motor output, 4, 7, 8, 18, 128
Munchausen-by-proxy syndrome, 152
Muscarinic effects, 155, 158, 160
Muscles
  involved in vomiting, 6–7, 8, 127–128. *See also* Contractions
  motion sickness and, 44
  poisoning and, 158, 161
  skeletal, and gastrointestinal motility, 67
  smooth gut, 61, 66, 67
Mushrooms, 144 (table), 146, 148, 154–155, 159–160
Mycardial infarction, 35, 147, 149, 152
Myoelectric activity, 73
Myoglobinuria, 147, 149
Myopathy, 65, 66, 67
Mysenteric plexus, 73

Nabilone, 117–118, 132
N-acetylcysteine, 148, 151
Naloxone, 2
Napthalene, 145 (table)
Naproxen, 145 (table)
Narcotic analgesics, 95 (table), 96, 97, 105
Nasogastric tube, 94, 151
Nasopharynx, 6
Nausea
  fasting, 70
  motion sickness and, 54–56
  phase, 127
  recurrent, 71
  See also Vomiting and nausea
Neurectomy, 31
Neuroanatomy, 1–8
Neuroendocrine reactions, 44, 47, 51–54
  treatment of, 57
Neurohypophysis, 44
Neuroinhibition, 7
Neurolabyrinthitis, 30, 33–35
Neurologic symptoms, 28, 30, 153
Neuromuscular disorders, 61
Neurons, 3, 4, 7, 8
Neuropathy, 65, 66
  poisoning as cause of, 153, 157
  types of, 67–68
Neuropeptide, 52
Neurotic reaction, 61. *See also* Psychogenic vomiting
Neurotransmitter receptors, 1, 5, 8, 129–130
Nicotine, 153, 158
Nitrous oxide, 97, 99, 103
  in oxygen and thiopental, 104–105
Nonapeptide, 54
Nonsteroidal anti-inflammatory agent, 144 (table), 146

Noradrenergic nervous system, 53
Norepinephrine, 44, 51
Nucleus tractus solitarius, 3, 5, 128
"Nutcracker esophagus," 64
Nutrition
  central parenteral, 74
  during pregnancy, 77, 80–81
  See also Diet; Malnutrition
Nystagmus, 29–30, 152
  Meniere's syndrome and, 32
  vertebrobasilar insufficiency and, 35

Obesity, 95 (table)
Obstruction (gastrointestinal), 71
  from inflammation or ulceration, 63
  mechanical, 61, 62, 143, 149–151
  pseudo-. *See* Intestinal pseudo-obstruction
  from scarring, 144
Ogilvie's syndrome, 65
Oils/lubricants, 144 (table)
Oliguria, 81
Ondansetron, 106–107, 119–120, 134
  in combination with other drugs, 137
Opioids, 53, 57, 97, 152
Optokinetic drum, 44, 46–50, 54, 56
Orchiopexy, 95
Organochlorines, 153, 158
Organophosphates, 153
Oropharyngeal nerve discharge, 7
Orthostatic hypotension, 68
Oscillipsia, 28
Otoliths, 45, 46
Otomastoiditis, 34
Oxalate, 145
Oxidizing agent, 145 (table)

Pain, 61, 62–63, 66
  in intestinal pseudo-obstruction, 73
  and postoperative nausea and vomiting, 95 (table)
  from toxins, 143–144, 149, 154–159
Pallor, 6
  and anticipatory nausea and vomiting, 19
  motion sickness and, 43
  vertigo and, 27
Pancreas, 6, 143, 147, 149
Pandysautonomia, 68
Paralysis, 155, 161
Paraquat, 144
Parasympathetic nervous system, 20
  motion sickness and, 50, 51, 54
  poisoning and, 158
Parathyroidism, 82
Paraventricular hypothalamic subnuclei, 3
Parenteral nutrition, 74
Paresthesia, 154–161
Parkinson's disease, 68
Paroxysmal positional nystagmus, 29–30
Pathogenic vomiting, 61
Pattern generator, 3–4, 128
  motion sickness and, 44, 55